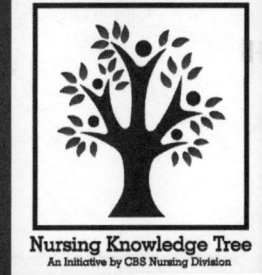

Practical Record Book of

Community Health Nursing-I

for GNM 1st Year Nursing Students

(AS per the New Syllabus of Indian Nursing Council for GNM)

Indu Rathore MSc (CHN)

Assistant Professor
Murari Lal Memorial School and College of Nursing
Solan, Himachal Pradesh, India

Foreword

Sushma Kumari Saini

CBSPD
Dedicated to Education

CBS Publishers & Distributors Pvt Ltd

• New Delhi • Bengaluru • Chennai • Kochi • Kolkata • Lucknow • Mumbai
• Hyderabad • Jharkhand • Nagpur • Patna • Pune • Uttarakhand

Practical Record Book of

Community Health Nursing-I

for GNM 1st Years Nursing Students

ISBN: 978-93-86827-07-4

Copyright © Author and Publishers

Reprint: 2025
Revise Reprint: 2020
First Edition: 2018

Published by **Satish Kumar Jain** and produced by **Varun Jain** for

CBS Publishers & Distributors Pvt Ltd

4819/XI Prahlad Street, 24 Ansari Road, Daryaganj, New Delhi 110 002, India.
Ph: +91-11-23289259, 23266861, 23266867   Website: www.cbspd.com
Fax: 011-23243014
e-mail: delhi@cbspd.com; cbspubs@airtelmail.in.

Corporate Office: 204 FIE, Industrial Area, Patparganj, Delhi 110 092
Ph: +91-11-4934 4934   Fax: 4934 4935
e-mail: feedback@cbspd.com; bhupesharora@cbspd.com

Branches

- **Bengaluru:** Seema House 2975, 17th Cross, K.R. Road, Banashankari 2nd Stage, Bengaluru 560 070, Karnataka
  Ph: +91-80-26771678/79   Fax: +91-80-26771680   e-mail: bangalore@cbspd.com
- **Chennai:** 7, Subbaraya Street, Shenoy Nagar, Chennai 600 030, Tamil Nadu
  Ph: +91-44-26680620, 26681266   Fax: +91-44-42032115   e-mail: chennai@cbspd.com
- **Kochi:** 68/1534, 35, 36-Power House Road, Opp. KSEB, Cochin-682018, Kochi, Kerala
  Ph: +91-484-4059061-65   Fax: +91-484-4059065   e-mail: kochi@cbspd.com
- **Kolkata:** Hind Ceramics Compound, 1st floor, 147, Nilganj Road, Belghoria, Kolkata-700056, West Bengal
  Ph: +033-2563-3055/56   e-mail: kolkata@cbspd.com
- **Lucknow:** Basement, Khushnuma Complex, 7-Meerabai Marg (Behind Jawahar Bhawan), Lucknow-226001, Uttar Pradesh
  Ph: +0522-4000032   e-mail: tiwari.lucknow@cbspd.com
- **Mumbai:** PWD Shed, Gala No. 25/26, Ramchandra Bhatt Marg, Next to J.J. Hospital Gate No. 2, Opp. Union Bank of India, Noor Baug, Mumbai-400009, Maharashtra
  Ph: +91-22-66661880/89   Fax: +91-22-24902342   e-mail: mumbai@cbspd.com

Representatives

- **Hyderabad**   +91-9885175004
- **Nagpur**   +91-9421945513
- **Pune**   +91-9623451994
- **Jharkhand**   +91-9811541605
- **Patna**   +91-9334159340
- **Uttarakhand** +91-9716462459

Printed at: Rashtriya printers Delhi-110095

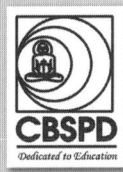
CBSPD
Dedicated to Education

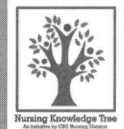
Nursing Knowledge Tree
An Initiative by CBS Nursing Division

CBS Nursing Knowledge Tree

Extends its Tribute to

Florence Nightingale

"

For glorifying the role of women as nurses,
For holding the title of " The Lady with the Lamp,"
For working tirelessly for humanity—
Florence Nightingale will always be
remembered for her
selfless and memorable services to the
human race.

"

Florence Nightingale
(May 1820 – August 1910)

Dedicated to

Almighty God
My Family
and
Dear Students
who have been inspiration for me at every step of my life.

Foreword

Community Health Nurses provide healthcare services to communities and improve their care accessibility. Key responsibilities of a community health nurse include: Identifying risk factors, improving access to services for under-served communities, promoting health care programs, providing direct care and screening services, educating people how to manage their conditions, performing immunizations, and ensuring maternal and child care. To fulfill these important roles, it is important for nursing students to learn skill in all these fields for which a comprehensive practical record book is very essential. I want to congratulate Ms Indu Rathore, Assistant Professor, Community Health Nursing, MLM School and College of Nursing, Solan (Himachal Pradesh) for bringing out such a comprehensive Practical Record Book of Community Health Nursing-I for GNM 1st Year Students.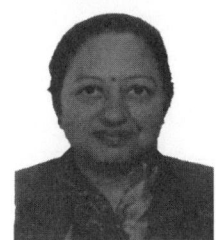

I personally liked the presentation of the book. It provides simple and systematic record for GNM Ist Year students. The nursing students guided by their teachers in various aspects are expected to maintain quality and standard for community experience based on requirements, which were established for every nursing institution. This record book will benefit the Community Health Nursing (CHN) students in gaining practical skills in documenting community profile, family nursing care plan, health and nutrition assessment of different age groups. It provides enough space for recording different procedures, health teaching, and visits to different health agencies. Enriched with reference notes, family folder and community survey proforma it inculcates better understanding of the practical aspects of CHN among nursing students. It also acts as guide for nursing teachers to teach and evaluate different aspects of community health nursing.

Annexures given at the end of book is a unique feature of this book. This gives a quick reference of different laboratory tests normal values, nutritive values for commonly used food items in India and recommended dietary allowances for various categories. For teachers, it has given sample evaluation proformas to evaluate each practical skill of student. Author has covered all the practical aspects of community health nursing in very easy to understand manner. A great deal of effort has been put into the format of the book to make it more user friendly. The entire book is prepared according to the current concepts of community health nursing. Upholds the latest syllabus and regulations of Indian Nursing Council.

I am sure this book will be proved as a boon for the nursing students and help them in strengthening their education, training and skill in performing their duties in implementing primary health care.

Sushma Kumari Saini
PhD (Public Administration), MSc Nursing (CHN)
Lecturer, National Institute of Nursing Education
PGIMER, Chandigarh, India

Preface

This Record Book is designed according to the community health nursing practical requirements of GNM, Ist Year students. Its main aim is to provide systematic, meaningful and comprehensive record of various activities and procedures carried out in a community setting. The record book is developed and updated according to latest syllabus prescribed by Indian Nursing Council, New Delhi.

The record book is prepared in a view to develop the standard format for conducting and writing the reports on community profile, family nursing care plans, health assessments of various age groups, health education plans, procedures or demonstrations using a standardized bag technique, A-V aid preparation, organization or participation in activities/clinics/camps, family folders and observation or orientation visits at health and welfare agencies. Further the evaluation proforma have been provided to maintain uniformity while evaluating nursing student's performance by the supervisors.

The special efforts have been taken to simplify the work and save time of supervisors or clinical instructors as well as nursing students. This record book serves as a valuable resource of logical, reliable and self-instructional formats to fulfill the community health nursing field requirements.

I hope that this record book will help the GNM Ist Year Students to gain knowledge and acquire competencies in community health nursing practice. I look forward for the valuable suggestions and reviews to make it more effective.

Indu Rathore

Acknowledgments

"When performance exceeds ambition, the overlap is called success"

First and foremost, I would like to thank the Lord for his grace and abundant blessings that I could complete this record book on time.

I express my sincere gratitude and I feel indebted to extend thanks to Mrs Shashi Sharma, Principal, MLM School and College of Nursing, Solan (Himachal Pradesh). Without her guidance and persistent help this work would not have been possible.

I am thankful to Mrs Neeti Sharma, Vice-principal, MLM School and College of Nursing, Solan (HP) for helping me to form valid concepts for this record book. Their deep insight and experience has given the present shape to my project.

I gratefully acknowledge Mr Nimit Gupta, Director, MLM School and College of Nursing, Solan (HP) for providing valuable assets, infrastructure and facilities throughout the writing period. He has all along been considerate, helpful and cordial despite his hectic schedule and official commitments.

I gratefully acknowledge the contribution all faculty members of MLM School and College of Nursing, Solan (HP) for their help and innumerable suggestions.

I will ever remain indebted to my family members—Father (Mr Shyam Babu Rathore), mother (Mrs Savitri Rathore), brother (Paurush) and sister (Neha), who always stood beside me through my tough times. They have been behind the scene, patiently encouraging and inspiring me.

Finally and perhaps most importantly, I would like to express my special appreciation to **Mr Satish Kumar Jain** (Chairman) and **Mr Varun Jain** (Managing Director), M/s CBS Publishers and Distributors Pvt Ltd for their wholehearted support in publication of this book. I also thank **Mr Bhupesh Aarora**, [Sr. Vice President – Publishing and Marketing (Health Sciences Division)] for providing me the platform to share knowledge and an opportunity to add to the existing knowledge of this field.

I sincerely thank the entire CBS team for bringing out the book with utmost care and attractive presentation. I would like to thank Ms Nitasha Arora (Assistant General Manager Publishing – Medical and Nursing), and Dr Anju Dhir (Sr. Product Manager and Medical Development Editor) for their publishing support. I would also extend my thanks to Ms Surbhi Gupta (Sr. English Editor), Mr Ashutosh Pathak (Sr. Proofreader cum Team Coordinator) and all the production team members for devoting laborious hours in designing and typesetting the book.

I extend my gratitude to all my students for their cooperation. My sincere thanks to all those who had directly and indirectly helped me in this endeavor.

From the Publisher's Desk

Dear Reader,

Nursing Education has a rich history, often characterized by traditional teaching techniques that have evolved over time. Primarily, teaching took place within classroom settings. Lectures, textbooks, and clinical rotations were the core teaching tools; and students majorly relied on textbooks by local or foreign publishers for quality education. However, today, technology has completely transformed the field of nursing education, making it an integral part of the curriculum. It has evolved to include a range of technological tools that enhance the learning experience and better prepare students for clinical practice.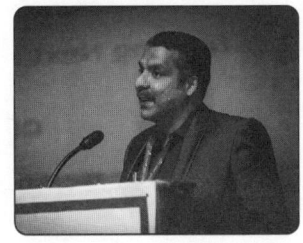

As publishers, we've been contributing to the field of Medical Science, Nursing and Allied Sciences and earned the trust of many. By supporting **Indian authors**, coupled with **nursing webinars and conferences**, we have paved an easier path for aspiring nurses, empowering them to excel in national and state level exams. With this, we're not only enhancing the quality of patient care but also enabling future nurses to adapt to new challenges and innovations in the rapidly evolving world of healthcare. Following the ideology of **Bringing learning to people instead of people going for learning**, so far, we've been doing our part by:

- Developing quality content by qualified and well-versed authors
- Building a strong community of faculty and students
- Introducing a smart approach with Digital/Hybrid Books, and
- Offering simulation Nursing Procedures, etc.

Innovative teaching methodologies, such as modern-age Phygital Books, have sparked the interest of the Next-Gen students in pursuing advanced education. The enhancement of educational standards through **Omnipresent Knowledge Sharing Platforms** has further facilitated learning, bridging the gap between doctors and nurses.

At Nursing Next Live, a sister concern of CBS Publishers & Distributors, we have long recognized the immense potential within the nursing field. Our journey in innovating nursing education has allowed us to make substantial and meaningful contributions. With the vision of strengthening learning at every stage, we have introduced several plans that cater to the specific needs of the students, including but not limited to **Plan UG** for undergraduates, **Plan MSc** for postgraduate aspirants, **Plan FDP** for upskilling faculties, **SDL** for integrated learning and **Plan NP** for bridging the gap between theoretical & practical learning. Additionally, we have successfully completed seven series of our **Target High** Book in a very short period, setting a milestone in the education industry. We have been able to achieve all this just with the sole vision of laying the foundation of diversified knowledge for all. With the rise of a new generation of educated, tech-savvy individuals, we anticipate even more remarkable advancements in the coming years.

We take immense pride in our achievements and eagerly look forward to the future, brimming with new opportunities for innovation, growth and collaborations with experienced minds such as yourself who can contribute to our mission as Authors, Reviewers and/or Faculties. Together, let's foster a generation of nurses who are confident, competent, and prepared to succeed in a technology-driven healthcare system.

Mr Bhupesh Aarora
(Sr Vice President – Publishing & Marketing)
bhupeshaarora@cbspd.com| +91 95553 53330

Syllabus for GNM Nursing

COMMUNITY HEALTH NURSING-I
PRACTICAL

Placement: First Year   **Time:** 336 Hours

Areas	Duration	Objectives	Skills	Assignments	Assessment methods
Community health Nursing - urban/rural	8 weeks	❑ Organize home visit ❑ Prepare bag and demonstrate bag technique. ❑ Build up and maintain rapport with family. ❑ Identify needs of community ❑ Practice procedure ❑ Make referrals. ❑ Plan and conduct health education on identified health needs. ❑ Set up clinics with help of staff. ❑ Maintain records and reports ❑ Collect and record vital health statistics. ❑ Learn about various organizations of community health importance. ❑ Health Assessment Family ❑ Identify the health needs of various age groups. ❑ Assess the environment ❑ Maintain family folders. ❑ Assessment nutritional needs ❑ Demonstrate different method of preparing food according to the nutritional need of family.	❑ Conducting Home visits. ❑ Nutritional assessment of individuals. ❑ Provide care at home as per Standing Orders/protocol. ❑ Conduct health education. ❑ Set up of different clinics. ❑ Maintain records and reports. ❑ Practice family Health nursing. ❑ Demonstrate different methods of preparation of meals.	❑ Daily Diary ❑ Health talk -2 ❑ Family care plan based on family study 2 ❑ Health assessment of an Individual -2 ❑ Community profile-2 ❑ Report of visit to water purification on plant, sewage plant, milk dairy, panchayat	❑ Assess clinical performance with rating scale. ❑ Evaluation of daily diary, health talk, family care plan, health assessment, community profile, observation report.

Contents

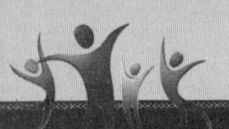

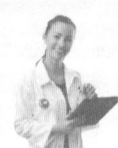

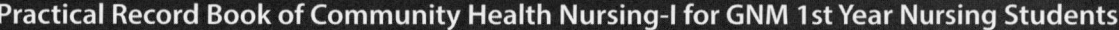
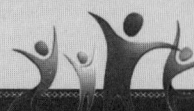
Practical Record Book Community Health Nursing-I for GNM 1st Year Nursing Students

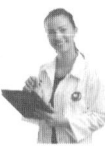

S. No.	Contents	No. of Records
1.	**Community Profile:** (Urban and Rural)	2
2.	**Family Nursing Care Plan:** (Urban and Rural)	2
3.	**Health Assessment:** (Urban and Rural)	2
4.	**Health Education:** (Urban and Rural)	2
5.	**Nutritional Assessment**	1
6.	**Nutritious Food Preparation/Cooking Demonstration**	1
7.	**Procedure Demonstration**	10
	❑ Bag Technique ❑ Vital Signs ❑ Urine Testing-Sugar/Albumin ❑ Oral Medication ❑ Minor Wound Dressing ❑ I.M./Subcutaneous Injection ❑ Steam Inhalation ❑ Collection of Specimen-Urine/Sputum ❑ Hydrotherapy ❑ Pediculosis Treatment	
8.	**Preparation of A-V Aids**—Charts, Flash Cards, Model, Pamphlet, Poster	5
9.	**Set up of Different Clinics**	4
	❑ Family Planning ❑ Immunization ❑ DOTS ❑ Any other (e.g. Malaria/Leprosy/ART)	
10.	**Observational Visits at Health and Welfare Agencies**	6
	❑ Water Purification Plant ❑ Sewage Purification Plant ❑ Milk Dairy ❑ Panchayat ❑ Any Other Community Organizations (e.g. Anganwadi, PHC-2 Additional)	
11.	**Home Visit and Family Folders**	

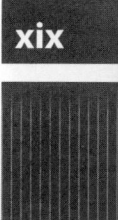

Student Profile

Paste Your Recent
Passport Size
Photograph in Uniform

Name of the Student: _____

Registration No./Enrolment No.: _____

Session/Batch: _____

Name of the Institution: _____

Name of the State Nursing Council:_____

Signature of Student   Signature of HOD   Signature of Principal

Date _____   Date _____   Date _____

Signature of:

Internal Examiner   External Examiner

Date _____   Date _____

Supplementary Examination

Signature of:

Internal Examiner   External Examiner

Date _____   Date _____

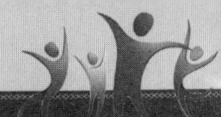
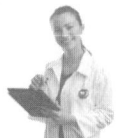

1. Community Profile

(Based on Community Identification and Vital Statistics Survey)

1.1. Urban

INTRODUCTION OF COMMUNITY

General Information

Village/Area Name: _____

Panchayat: _____

Block: _____

Tehsil/Taluka: _____

District: _____

Total population: _____

Total Families: _____

Nearby Health Care Facilities [Name and its distance (in km) from the community area]

District Hospital: _____

Government Maternity Hospital (if any): _____

Mission Hospital (if any): _____

Total Private Hospitals: _____

Subcenter: _____

Primary Health Center: _____

Community Health Center: _____

Indigenous Medicine (Hospital/Clinic/Dispensary)

- Ayurveda: _____
- Yoga: _____
- Naturopathy: _____
- Unani: _____
- Siddha: _____
- Homeopathy: _____
- If other, Specify: _____

Non-Governmental Organizations/Voluntary Health Organizations

- Orphan Age Children: _____
- Physically Challenged: _____
- Visually Challenged: _____

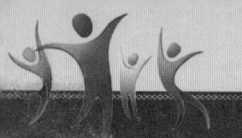

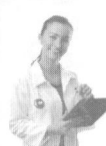

- Mentally Challenged: _____
- Hearing Challenged: _____
- Women: _____
- Elderly: _____
- Youth Welfare: _____
- Other: _____

Social Agencies

- Post Office: _____
- Bank: _____
- Police Station: _____

Religious Place

- Temple: _____
- Mosque: _____
- Gurudwara: _____
- Church: _____
- If Others, Specify: _____

Education Facilities

Government

- Anganwadis: _____
- Balwadis: _____
- Primary School: _____
- Elementary School: _____
- Secondary School: _____
- Senior Secondary School: _____
- UG Institutions: _____
- PG Institutions: _____

Private

- Primary School: _____
- Elementary School: _____
- Secondary School: _____
- Senior Secondary School: _____
- UG Institutions: _____
- PG Institutions: _____

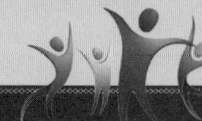

Recreation Facilities

- Common Market Place: _____
- Playgrounds: _____
- Public Gardens: _____
- Cinema Halls: _____
- Clubs: _____
- Public Library: _____
- Fairs: _____
- Festivals: _____

Communication Facilities

- Post Office: _____
- Public Telephone Booths: _____
- Computer Center with Internet Facility: _____
- Traditional Media (Puppets, Folk Dance etc.): _____

Transport Facilities

- Railway Station: _____
- Bus Stand: _____
- Auto Stand: _____
- Taxi Stand: _____
- Airport: _____

Facilities for the Disposal of Dead Bodies

_____
_____
_____
_____

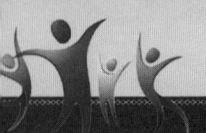
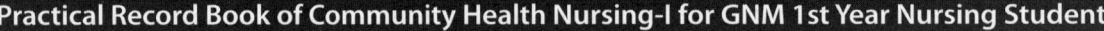
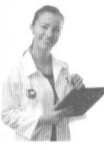

SOCIODEMOGRAPHIC DATA

N =

S. No.	Criteria	Sociodemographic Characteristics	n (%)
1.	Age Group	Infant (1–12 months) Under five children (1–5 years) School going (6–12 years) Adolescent (13–17 years) Early adult (18–45 years) Late adult (46–59 years) Geriatric (60 years and above)	
2.	Sex	Male Female Transgender	
3.	Religion*	Hindu Muslim Christian Sikh Others, Specify _____	
4.	Caste	General OBC SC ST	
5.	Education**	Illiterate Able to read and write Primary Up to 8th class Up to 10th Up to 12th Graduate Postgraduate PhD/M.Phil Others, Specify _____	
6.	Marital status	Married Single/Unmarried Widow	
7.	Type of family	Nuclear Joint Separated	
8.	Family Size	2–4 5–8 9 and above	
9.	Occupation	Employed—Government Job Private Job Unemployed Retired Daily wage workers Homemaker	
10.	Total family income (₹)	Up to 10,000 10,000-20,000 20,000 and above	

*Other religion _____   **Other educational qualification _____

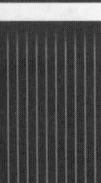

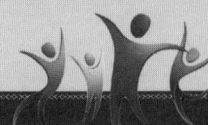

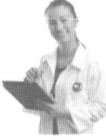

PHYSICAL CHARACTERISTICS OF AREA (MAP)

Keys

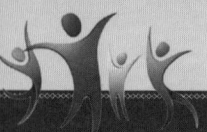

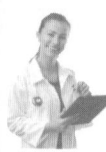

HOUSING STANDARDS

N =

S. No.	Criteria	Characteristics	n (%)
1.	Ownership of house	Rent Own	
2.	Type of house	Pucca Semi pucca Katcha	
3.	Number of living room per House	1–2 3–4 4 and above	

4.	Bathroom	Not available
		Available - Own
		          Public
		Hygiene - Hygienic
		          Unhygienic	

5.	Latrine	Not available
		Available - Own
		          Public
		Hygiene - Hygienic
		          Unhygienic	

6.	Electricity	Not available Available	
7.	Water Supply*	Tap Well Lake/pond Others, Specify _____	
8.	Kitchen **	Separate Corner of the room Others, Specify _____	
9.	Type of fuel used***	LPG Electricity Kerosene Wood Others, Specify _____	

*Other water supply source _____   **Other kitchen _____

***Other fuel used _____

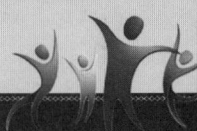

HOUSING ENVIRONMENT AND SANITATION

N =

S. No.	Criteria	Characteristics	n (%)
1.	Modern sanitation facility	Drainage system	
		Sewage system	
2.	Drainage system	Closed	
		Open	
3.	Refuse disposal	Open dumping	
		Composting	
		Burning	
		Municipality collection/community bins	
4.	Domestic animal*	Not present	
		Present - Dog	
		Cat	
		Buffalo	
		Cow	
		Goat	
		Others, Specify _____	
5.	Cattle shed (for the house with domestic animal)	Yes	
		No	
6.	Domestic birds/poultry**	Not present	
		Present - Hen/Cock	
		Parrot	
		Others, Specify _____	
7.	Poultry shed/cage (for the house with poultry)	Yes	
		No	
8.	Rodents	Not present	
		Yes - Rat	
		Others, Specify _____	
9.	Insects	Not present	
		Yes - Mosquitoes	
		Flies	
		Ticks	
		Others, Specify _____	
10.	Street animals	Not present	
		Yes - Dogs	
		Cats	
		Cows	
		Others, Specify _____	

*Other domestic animals _____

**Other domestic birds _____

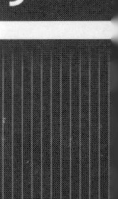

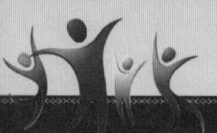
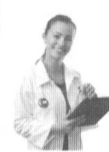

FAMILY PLANNING STATUS

N =

S. No.	Methods adopted for Family Planning		n (%)
1.	Temporary methods	Condoms	
		Oral Contraceptive Pills (OCP)	
		Copper-T (Cu-T)	
		Injectables	
		Subdermal implants	
2.	Permanent methods	Tubectomy	
		Vasectomy	
3.	Not adopting any family planning method		

COMMON HEALTH PROBLEMS

N =

S. No.	Health Problems	n (%)
1.	Communicable diseases	
2.	Noncommunicable diseases	
3.	Nutritional problems	
4.	Mental health problems	
5.	Acute problems	
6.	Chronic problems	

VITAL STATISTICS

1. Crude Birth Rate

$$\text{Crude Birth Rate} = \frac{\text{No. of live birth during the year}}{\text{Estimated mid-year population}} \times 1000$$

Crude Birth Rate = _____

2. Crude Death Rate

$$\text{Crude Death Rate} = \frac{\text{No. of deaths during the year}}{\text{Estimated mid-year population}} \times 1000$$

Crude Death Rate = _____

3. Infant Mortality Rate

$$\text{Infant Mortality Rate} = \frac{\text{No. of deaths under one year of age}}{\text{Total live births in the same year}} \times 1000$$

Infant Mortality Rate = _____

4. Neonatal Mortality Rate

$$\text{Neonatal Mortality Rate} = \frac{\text{No. of deaths of children less than 28 days in a year}}{\text{Total live births in the same year}} \times 1000$$

Neonatal Mortality Rate = _____

5. Stillbirth Rate

$$\text{Stillbirth Rate} = \frac{\text{No. of Stillbirths in a year}}{\text{Total live births and Stillbirths in the same year}} \times 1000$$

Stillbirth Rate = _____

6. Maternal Mortality Rate

$$\text{Maternal Mortality Rate} = \frac{\text{Total No. of female deaths due to complications of pregnancy, child birth or within 42 days of delivery during a given year}}{\text{Total number of live births in the same year}} \times 1000$$

Maternal Mortality Rate = _____

7. General Fertility Rate

$$\text{General Fertility Rate} = \frac{\text{No. of live births in area during the year}}{\text{Mid-year female population age group (15–49) in the same year}} \times 1000$$

General Fertility Rate = _____

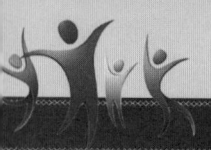
ONGOING COMMUNITY HEALTH PROGRAMMES

(Communicable/noncommunicable diseases/others)

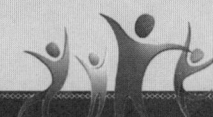
ONGOING SOCIAL WELFARE/HEALTH SCHEMES

Physically/Visually/Mentally/Hearing Challenged

_____

_____

_____

_____

Women (Antenatal/Postnatal/Widow)

_____

_____

_____

_____

Children

_____

_____

_____

Adolescent Girls

_____

_____

_____

_____

BPL Families

_____

_____

_____

Elderly

_____

_____

_____

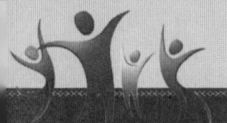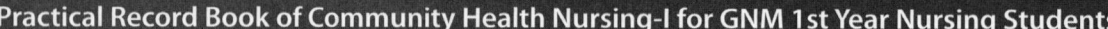

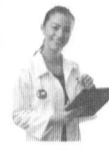

LIST OF COMMUNITY LEADERS

Departments	Designations	Names	Addresses	Contact number
FORMAL LEADERS				
Political system	MLA			
	MP			
	Representative of women			
	Representative of SC/ST			
	Trade Union Leaders			
Gram panchayat	President (Pradhan/Sarpanch)			
	Vice President/Panchayat secretary (Uppradhan/Upsarpanch)			
Ward	Ward member (councilor)			
Health	Health worker (Female)			
	Health worker (Male)			
	Anganwadi worker			
INFORMAL LEADERS				
School	School teacher			
Society	Social worker			
	Retired person			
Others				

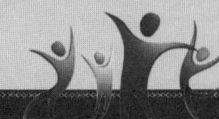

IDENTIFIED COMMUNITY HEALTH NEEDS

_____
_____
_____
_____
_____
_____
_____
_____
_____
_____
_____
_____
_____
_____

PLANNING/NURSING INTERVENTIONS

_____
_____
_____
_____
_____
_____
_____
_____
_____

_____

Signature of Student

_____

Signature of Supervisor

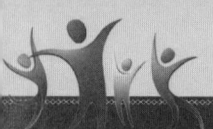
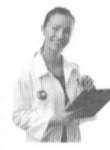

1.2. Rural

INTRODUCTION OF COMMUNITY

General Information

Village/Area Name: _____

Panchayat: _____

Block: _____

Tehsil/Taluka: _____

District: _____

Total population: _____

Total Families: _____

Nearby Health Care Facilities [Name and its distance (in km) from the community area]

District Hospital: _____

Government Maternity Hospital (if any): _____

Mission Hospital (if any): _____

Total Private Hospitals: _____

Subcenter: _____

Primary Health Center: _____

Community Health Center: _____

Indigenous Medicine (Hospital/Clinic/Dispensary)

- Ayurveda: _____
- Yoga: _____
- Naturopathy: _____
- Unani: _____
- Siddha: _____
- Homeopathy: _____
- If other, Specify: _____

Non-Governmental Organizations/Voluntary Health Organizations

- Orphan Age Children: _____
- Physically Challenged: _____
- Visually Challenged: _____
- Mentally Challenged: _____

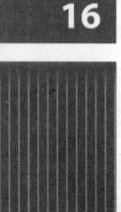

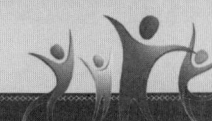

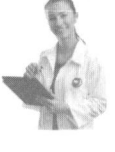

- Hearing Challenged: _____
- Women: _____
- Elderly: _____
- Youth Welfare: _____
- Other: _____

Social Agencies

- Post Office: _____
- Bank:_____
- Police Station: _____

Religious Place

- Temple: _____
- Mosque: _____
- Gurudwara: _____
- Church: _____
- If Others, Specify: _____

Education Facilities

Government

- Anganwadis: _____
- Balwadis: _____
- Primary School: _____
- Elementary School: _____
- Secondary School: _____
- Senior Secondary School: _____
- UG Institutions: _____
- PG Institutions: _____

Private

- Primary School: _____
- Elementary School: _____
- Secondary School: _____
- Senior Secondary School: _____
- UG Institutions: _____
- PG Institutions: _____

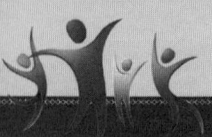

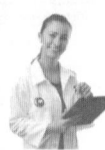

Recreation Facilities

- Common Market Place: _____
- Playgrounds: _____
- Public Gardens: _____
- Cinema Halls: _____
- Clubs: _____
- Public Library: _____
- Fairs: _____
- Festivals: _____

Communication Facilities

- Post Office: _____
- Public Telephone Booths: _____
- Computer Center with Internet Facility: _____
- Traditional Media (Puppets, Folk Dance etc.): _____

Transport Facilities

- Railway Station: _____
- Bus Stand: _____
- Auto Stand: _____
- Taxi Stand: _____
- Airport: _____

Facilities for the Disposal of Dead Bodies

_____

_____

_____

_____

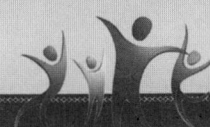

SOCIODEMOGRAPHIC DATA

N =

S. No.	Criteria	Sociodemographic Characteristics	n (%)
1.	Age group	Infant (1–12 months) Under five children (1–5 years) School going (6–12 years) Adolescent (13–17 years) Early adult (18–45 years) Late adult (46–59 years) Geriatric (60 years and above)	
2.	Sex	Male Female Transgender	
3.	Religion*	Hindu Muslim Christian Sikh Others, Specify _____	
4.	Caste	General OBC SC ST	
5.	Education**	Illiterate Able to read and write Primary Up to 8th class Up to 10th Up to 12th Graduate Postgraduate PhD/M.Phil Others, Specify _____	
6.	Marital status	Married Single/Unmarried Widow	
7.	Type of family	Nuclear Joint Separated	
8.	Family size	2–4 5–8 9 and above	
9.	Occupation	Employed—Government Job Private Job Unemployed Retired Daily wage workers Homemaker	
10.	Total family income (₹)	Up to 10,000 10,000-20,000 20,000 and above	

*Other religion _____ **Other educational qualification _____

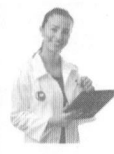

PHYSICAL CHARACTERISTICS OF AREA (MAP)

Keys

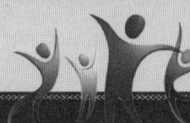

HOUSING STANDARDS

N =

S. No.	Criteria	Characteristics	n (%)
1.	Ownership of house	Rent Own	
2.	Type of house	Pucca Semi pucca Katcha	
3.	Number of living room per House	1–2 3–4 4 and above	
4.	Bathroom	Not available Available - Own Public Hygiene - Hygienic Unhygienic	
5.	Latrine	Not available Available - Own Public Hygiene - Hygienic Unhygienic	
6.	Electricity	Not available Available	
7.	Water Supply*	Tap Well Lake/pond Others, Specify _____	
8.	Kitchen **	Separate Corner of the room Others, Specify _____	
9.	Type of fuel used***	LPG Electricity Kerosene Wood Others, Specify _____	

*Other water supply source _____ **Other kitchen _____

***Other fuel used _____

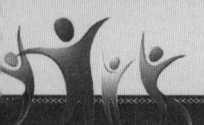 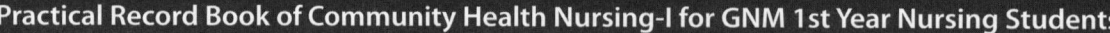

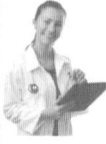

HOUSING ENVIRONMENT AND SANITATION

N =

S. No.	Criteria	Characteristics	n (%)
1.	Modern sanitation facility	Drainage system	
		Sewage system	
2.	Drainage system	Closed	
		Open	
3.	Refuse disposal	Open dumping	
		Composting	
		Burning	
		Municipality collection/community bins	
4.	Domestic animal*	Not present	
		Present - Dog	
		Cat	
		Buffalo	
		Cow	
		Goat	
		Others, Specify _____	
5.	Cattle shed (for the house with domestic animal)	Yes	
		No	
6.	Domestic birds/poultry**	Not present	
		Present - Hen/Cock	
		Parrot	
		Others, Specify _____	
7.	Poultry shed/cage (for the house with poultry)	Yes	
		No	
8.	Rodents	Not present	
		Yes – Rat	
		Others, Specify _____	
9.	Insects	Not present	
		Yes – Mosquitoes	
		Flies	
		Ticks	
		Others, Specify _____	
10.	Street animals	Not present	
		Yes – Dogs	
		Cats	
		Cows	
		Others, Specify _____	

*Other domestic animals _____

**Other domestic birds _____

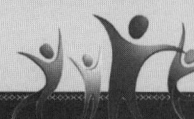

FAMILY PLANNING STATUS

N =

S. No.	Methods adopted for Family Planning		n (%)
1.	Temporary methods	Condoms	
		Oral Contraceptive Pills (OCP)	
		Copper-T (Cu-T)	
		Injectables	
		Subdermal implants	
2.	Permanent methods	Tubectomy	
		Vasectomy	
3.	Not adopting any family planning method		

COMMON HEALTH PROBLEMS

N =

S. No.	Health Problems	n (%)
1.	Communicable diseases	
2.	Noncommunicable diseases	
3.	Nutritional problems	
4.	Mental health problems	
5.	Acute problems	
6.	Chronic problems	

VITAL STATISTICS

1. Crude Birth Rate

$$\text{Crude Birth Rate} = \frac{\text{No. of live birth during the year}}{\text{Estimated mid-year population}} \times 1000$$

Crude Birth Rate = _____

2. Crude Death Rate

$$\text{Crude Death Rate} = \frac{\text{No. of deaths during the year}}{\text{Estimated mid-year population}} \times 1000$$

Crude Death Rate = _____

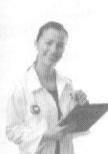

3. Infant Mortality Rate

$$\text{Infant Mortality Rate} = \frac{\text{No. of deaths under one year of age}}{\text{Total live births in the same year}} \times 1000$$

Infant Mortality Rate = _____

4. Neonatal Mortality Rate

$$\text{Neonatal Mortality Rate} = \frac{\text{No. of deaths of children less than 28 days in a year}}{\text{Total live births in the same year}} \times 1000$$

Neonatal Mortality Rate = _____

5. Stillbirth Rate

$$\text{Stillbirth Rate} = \frac{\text{No. of Stillbirths in a year}}{\text{Total live births and Stillbirths in the same year}} \times 1000$$

Stillbirth Rate = _____

6. Maternal Mortality Rate

$$\text{Maternal Mortality Rate} = \frac{\text{Total No. of female deaths due to complications of pregnancy, child birth or within 42 days of delivery during a given year}}{\text{Total number of live births in the same year}} \times 1000$$

Maternal Mortality Rate = _____

7. General Fertility Rate

$$\text{General Fertility Rate} = \frac{\text{No. of live births in area during the year}}{\text{Mid-year female population age group (15–49) in the same year}} \times 1000$$

General Fertility Rate = _____

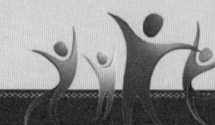

ONGOING COMMUNITY HEALTH PROGRAMMES

(Communicable/noncommunicable diseases/others)

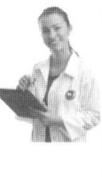

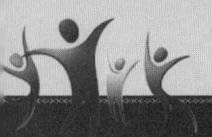
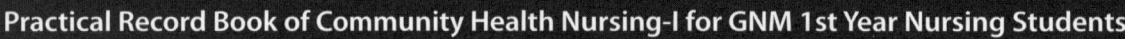
ONGOING SOCIAL WELFARE/HEALTH SCHEMES

Physically/Visually/Mentally/Hearing Challenged

_____

_____

_____

_____

Women (Antenatal/Postnatal/Widow)

_____

_____

_____

_____

Children

_____

_____

_____

Adolescent Girls

_____

_____

_____

_____

BPL Families

_____

_____

_____

Elderly

_____

_____

_____

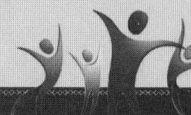
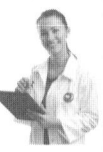

LIST OF COMMUNITY LEADERS

Departments	Designations	Names	Addresses	Contact numbers
FORMAL LEADERS				
Political system	MLA			
	MP			
	Representative of women			
	Representative of SC/ST			
	Trade Union Leaders			
Gram panchayat	President (Pradhan/Sarpanch)			
	Vice President/Panchayat secretary (Uppradhan/Upsarpanch)			
Ward	Ward member (councilor)			
Health	Health worker (Female)			
	Health worker (Male)			
	Anganwadi worker			
INFORMAL LEADERS				
School	School teacher			
Society	Social worker			
	Retired person			
Others				

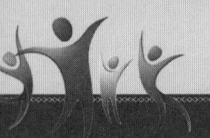
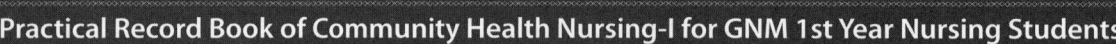

IDENTIFIED COMMUNITY HEALTH NEEDS

_____
_____
_____
_____
_____
_____
_____
_____
_____
_____
_____
_____
_____
_____
_____
_____

PLANNING/NURSING INTERVENTIONS

_____
_____
_____
_____
_____
_____
_____
_____
_____
_____
_____

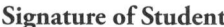

Signature of Student

Signature of Supervisor

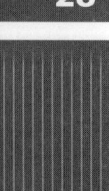

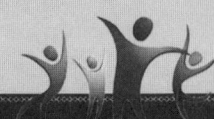

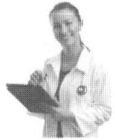

2. Family Nursing Care Plan

2.1. Urban

INTRODUCTION OF THE FAMILY

General Information

Name of Head of the Family: _____

Address: _____

Religion—Hindu/Muslims/Sikh/Christian/Others: _____
_____

Caste—GEN/SC/ST/OBC: _____

Occupation of the Head of the Family—Unemployed/
Government/Private Job/Self-Employed/Daily Wage Worker/
Homemaker/Others: _____

Language Known—Hindi/English/Others: _____

Family Size (Total Members): _____

Family type—Nuclear/Joint: _____

Ownership of House—Own/Rented: _____

Monthly Family Income: ₹: _____

Family Income per Capita: ₹: _____

Date of Starting: _____

Date of Ending: _____

FAMILY COMPOSITION AND CHARACTERISTICS

S. No.	Name of the family members	Relationship with head of the family	Date of birth/ sex (Male-M/ Female-F/ Transgender-T)	Marital status (Unmarried/ married)	Educa-tional status	Occu-pation	Monthly income (₹)	Dietary habits (Veg/ non-veg)	Addiction (Smoking Alcohol/ Drugs/ Others)	Health status (Healthy/ unhealthy)
1.										
2.										
3.										
4.										
5.										
6.										
7.										
8.										

Family Tree/Genogramme

Key

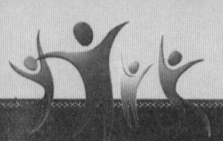

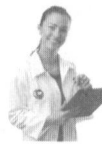

AVAILABILITY OF HEALTH CARE/SOCIAL/EDUCATIONAL FACILITIES

Facilities	Yes/No (If yes, specify name and distance from the house)
Nearby Health Care Facilities	
District hospital	
Government maternity hospital (if any)	
Private hospitals	
Subcenter	
Primary health center	
Community health center	
Indigenous medicine (hospital/clinic/dispensary)	
• Ayurveda	
• Yoga	
• Naturopathy	
• Unani	
• Siddha	
• Homeopathy	
• If other, specify	
Non-Governmental Organizations/Voluntary Health Organizations	
• Orphan age children	
• Physically challenged	
• Visually challenged	
• Mentally challenged	
• Hearing challenged	
• Women	
• Elderly	
• Youth welfare	
• Other	
Social Agencies	
• Post office	
• Bank	
• Police station	
Education Facilities **Government**	
• Anganwadis	
• Balwadis	
• Primary school	
• Elementary school	
• Secondary school	
• Senior secondary school	
• UG Institutions	
• PG institutions	
Private	
• Primary school	
• Elementary school	
• Secondary school	
• Senior secondary school	
• UG Institutions	
• PG institutions	

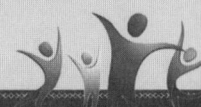

AVAILABILITY OF RECREATION/COMMUNICATION/TRANSPORT/RELIGIOUS FACILITIES

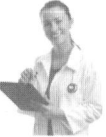

Facilities	Yes/No (If yes, specify name and distance from the house)
Recreation Facilities	
• Nearby market	
• Playgrounds	
• Public Gardens	
• Cinema halls	
• Clubs	
• Public library	
• Fairs	
• Festivals	
Communication Facilities	
• Telephone connection	
• Mobile phone	
• Internet facility	
• Letters	
Transport facilities	
• Bus	
• Auto rickshaw	
• Taxi	
• Four wheeler	
• Two wheeler	
• Train	
• Airway	
Religious Places	
• Temple	
• Mosque	
• Gurudwara	
• Church	

Sketch of House

(Draw a sketch of the house showing location of rooms, doors, windows, entrance of the house, drinking water source, toilet and kitchen)

Key

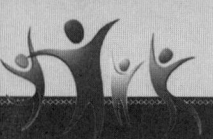
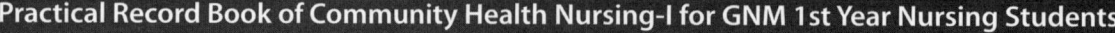
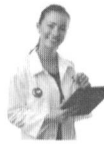

HOUSING STANDARDS AND ENVIRONMENTAL CONDITIONS

Characteristics	Parameters
Type of house	Pucca/Semi pucca/Katcha
Site	Elevated from surroundings/depressed from surroundings
Total number of living room	1/2/3/4/5/6/7/8/ _____
Space per person	Adequate (1 room -2 persons, 2 rooms -3 persons, 3 rooms – 5 persons, 4 rooms -7 persons, 5 or more rooms - 10 persons (additional 2 for each further room Inadequate (if above criteria is not fulfilled)
Ventilation	Adequate (doors and windows facing each other in each room) Inadequate (doors and windows not facing each other in each room)
Bathroom 　Hygiene	Not available/If available—Own/Public Hygienic/Unhygienic
Wall	Plastered or Cemented/Tiled/Wooden/Unplastered/Mud//Others, specify _____
Roof 　Height 　Painting	 Less than 10 feet/More than 10 feet Light colored/Dark colored
Day light	Adequate (Able to read the small fonts of newspaper inside the room during the day without any artificial lighting) Inadequate (Not able to read the small fonts of newspaper inside the room during the day without any artificial lighting)
Latrine 　Hygiene	Not available/If available—Own/Public Hygienic/Unhygienic
Electricity	Not available/Available
Drinking water supply	Tap/Well/Lake/Pond/Others, specify _____
Kitchen	Separate/Corner of the room/Others, specify _____
Type of fuel used	LPG/Electricity/Kerosene/Wood/Others, specify _____
Open space around the house	Absent/Present
Stagnant water around the house	Absent/Present
Street road	Tar/Cement/Mud/Others
Street light	Absent/Present
Modern sanitation facility 　Drainage system 　Sewage system	 Yes/No Yes/No
Drainage system	Closed/Open
Refuse disposal	Open dumping/Composting/Burning/Municipality collection/Community bins/Others, specify _____
Domestic animal	Absent/If present—Dog/Cow/Buffalo/Goat/Camel/Others, specify _____
Separate cattle shed (for the house with domestic animals)	Yes/No
Domestic birds/Poultry	Absent/If present—Hen/Cock/Parrot/Others, specify _____
Separate poultry shed/cage (for the house with domestic birds)	Yes/No
Rodents	Absent/If present—Rat/Others, specify _____
Street animals	Absent/If present—Dogs/Cats/Cows/Others, specify _____
Insect vectors	Absent/If present—Mosquitoes/Flies/Ticks/Others, specify _____

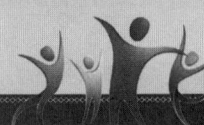
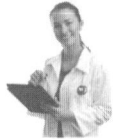

SOCIOECONOMIC STATUS

Social class/Socioeconomic status (according to rural/urban socioeconomic scale, Refer to Annexures)

_____

VULNERABLE/TARGET GROUPS IN THE FAMILY

Total eligible couples _____   Children (0–1 years) _____   Adolescent Girls _____

Total postnatal mothers _____   Children (1–3 years) _____   Elderly (above 60 years) _____

Total antenatal mothers _____   Children (3–5 years) _____   Other, specify _____

MONTHLY FAMILY BUDGET

Income			Expenditure		
Sources	**Income (In ₹)**	**Income (In Percentage)**	**Sources**	**Expenditure (In ₹)**	**Expenditure (In Percentage)**
Salary			House rent		
Rent			Education		
Agriculture			Food		
Animals			Fuel (LPG)		
Pension			Fuel (Petrol/Diesel)		
Stipend			Clothing		
Part time business			Entertainment		
Others			Electricity		
			Water		
			Property taxes		
			Telephone/Internet		
			Transportation		
			Health		
			Festival		
			Saving		
			Insurance		
			Others		
Total (₹)			**Total (₹)**		

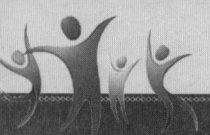
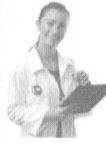

FAMILY DIETARY PATTERN

Food groups	Food items	Food consumption (Yes/No)	Frequency of consumption (Servings per day or per week)	Method/Form of food preparation (Boiling/steaming/raw/ pressure cooking/ frying/germination, etc.)	Method of food storage at home (Hygienic-H/ Unhygienic-U)
Energy giving foods	Rice				
	Wheat				
	Tubers				
	Edible oil				
	Ghee				
	Butter				
Body building foods	Meat				
	Fish				
	Poultry				
	Eggs				
	Pulses				
Protective foods	Vegetables				
	Fruits				
	Milk & milk products				
Beverages	Tea				
	Coffee				
	Water				
Others	Junk food				

SOCIOCULTURAL ASPECTS

Menstruation _____

_____

_____

_____

_____

_____

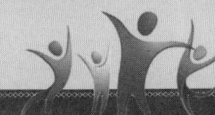

Antenatal Care _____

_____

_____

_____

_____

_____

Child Birth _____

_____

_____

_____

_____

_____

Postnatal Care _____

_____

_____

_____

_____

_____

Care of Sick _____

_____

_____

_____

_____

_____

_____

Food Consumption _____

_____

_____

_____

_____

_____

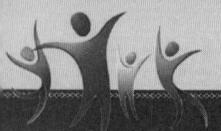
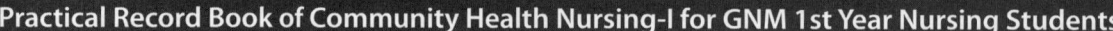
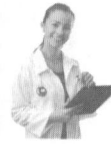

FAMILY PLANNING STATUS (ELIGIBLE COUPLE)

S. No.	Name of the eligible couple (Mr. _____ Mrs _____)	Age (yrs.)/ Sex (Male-M Female-F)	Family planning practice (a) Yes (b) No	If yes, then							Month and year of adoption/ duration of use
				Temporary family planning method					Permanent family planning method		
				Condom	Oral pills	Copper-T	Inject able	Implant	Tubectomy	Vasectomy	
1.											
2.											
3.											
4.											

IMMUNIZATION STATUS

Age Group	Weeks/ Months/Years	Current Vaccine Under UIP (2017)	Child Name/Vaccines/Date of Administration (DOA)					
			Child -1 _____		Child -2 _____		Child -3 _____	
			Vaccines	DOA	Vaccines	DOA	Vaccines	DOA
Infant	At birth	BCG, OPV-0, Hep-B birth dose						
	6 weeks	OPV-1, Rota-1, Pentavalent-1, IPV-1, PCV-1						
	10 weeks	OPV-2, Rota-2, Pentavalent-2						
	14 weeks	OPV-3, Rota-3, Pentavalent-3, IPV-2, PCV-2						
	9 months	MR/Measles-1, Vit-A*, JE-1#, PCV-Booster						
Under five children	16–24 months	DPT-Booster-1, OPV-Booster, MR/Measles-2, JE-2#						
School going	5–6 Years	DPT-Booster -2						
Adolescent	10 years	TT-1						
	16 years	TT-2						
Pregnancy		TT-1						
		TT-2						

*Vitamin A to be given every 6 months till five years of age and a separate chart is given below for documentation. #JE vaccine given in selected districts. **BCG:** Bacillus Calmette-Guerin; **Pentavalent [DPT:** diphtheria-pertussis-tetanus; **Hep B:** Hepatitis B; **Hib:** Haemophilus influenzae type b]; **JE:** Japanese Encephalitis; **MR/Measles/MMR:** Measles Mumps rubella; **OPV:** oral polio vaccine; **TT:** tetanus toxoid; **IPV:** inactivated poliovirus vaccine. **Rota-** Rotavirus vaccine, **PCV:** Pneumonia; Additional _____

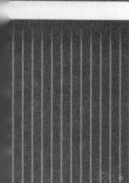

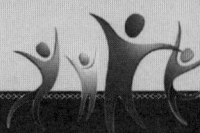
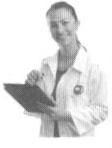

Age (in months) →		9	18	24	30	36	42	48	54	60
Dose →		1st	2nd	3rd	4th	5th	6th	7th	8th	9th
Vitamin-A Solution (DOA)	Child-1 _____									
	Child-2 _____									
	Child-3 _____									

VITAL EVENTS IN THE FAMILY DURING THE LAST ONE YEAR

Birth (if any)

S. No.	Name	Date of birth	Sex	Parents name	Place of birth	Birth registration-Yes/No
1.						
2.						
3.						

Death (if any)

S. No.	Name	Date of death	Age/Sex	Cause of death	Place of death	Death registration-Yes/No
1.						
2.						
3.						

Marriage (if any)

S. No.	Name of the couple	Age		Date of marriage	Marriage registration-Yes/No
		Wife	Husband		
1.					
2.					
3.					

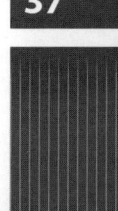

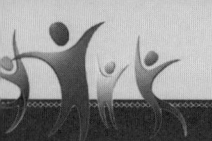

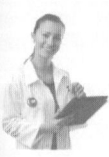

Family Health Profile

Instructions

1. Select a key case(s) from the assigned family—elderly/adult/adolescent/antenatal/postnatal/newborn/under five/physically challenged/sick/vulnerable or specific group as per assigned family priority health need.

2. Write the selected family member(s)—identification data, health history, specific physical assessment, lab investigations (if any), medications, diet chart, identified health needs/problems and disease condition (book picture)

3. Eight blank pages are provided here. If more details are required, paste the additional pages in the record book.

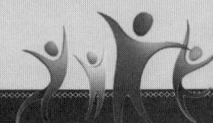

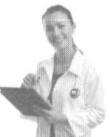

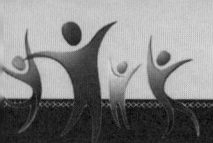

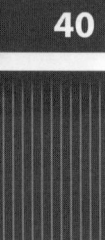

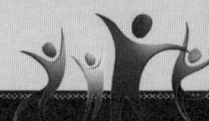
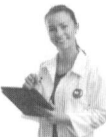

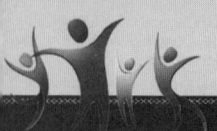

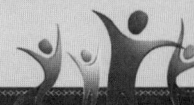

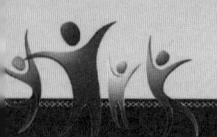
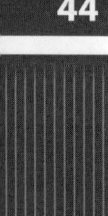

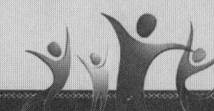

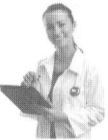

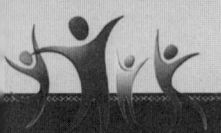

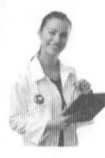

Instructions
1. Identify the family health needs, prioritize them, formulate the possible nursing diagnosis and write the nursing care plan.
2. If more details are required, paste the additional pages in the record book.

Identified Health Problems/Needs

_____
_____
_____
_____
_____
_____

Prioritization of Health Problems/Needs

_____
_____
_____
_____
_____
_____

Priority Nursing Diagnosis

_____
_____
_____
_____
_____
_____
_____
_____
_____
_____
_____

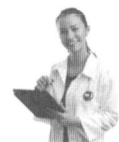

FAMILY HEALTH NURSING CARE PLAN

Assessment	Diagnosis	Goal/ Objective	Planning	Implementation	Evaluation

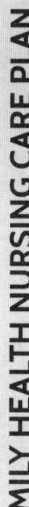

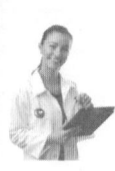

FAMILY HEALTH NURSING CARE PLAN

Assessment	Diagnosis	Goal/Objective	Planning	Implementation	Evaluation

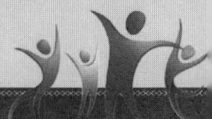

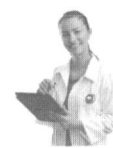

FAMILY HEALTH NURSING CARE PLAN

Assessment	Diagnosis	Goal/Objective	Planning	Implementation	Evaluation

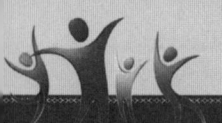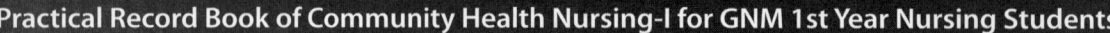

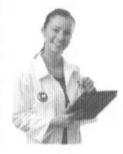

FAMILY HEALTH NURSING CARE PLAN

Assessment	Diagnosis	Goal/ Objective	Planning	Implementation	Evaluation

HEALTH EDUCATION

REFERENCES

Signature of Student

Signature of Supervisor

50

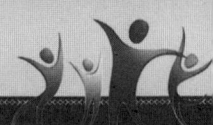

2.2. Rural

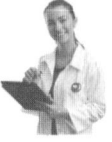

INTRODUCTION OF THE FAMILY

General Information

Name of Head of the Family: _____

Address: _____

Religion—Hindu/Muslims/Sikh/Christian/Others: _____
_____

Caste—GEN/SC/ST/OBC: _____

Occupation of the Head of the Family—Unemployed/ Government/Private Job/Self-Employed/Daily Wage Worker/ Homemaker/Others: _____

Language Known—Hindi/English/Others: _____

Family Size (Total Members): _____

Family type—Nuclear/Joint: _____

Ownership of House—Own/Rented: _____

Monthly Family Income: ₹: _____

Family Income per Capita: ₹: _____

Date of Starting: _____

Date of Ending: _____

FAMILY COMPOSITION AND CHARACTERISTICS

S. No.	Name of the family members	Relationship with head of the family	Date of birth/ sex (Male-M/ Female-F/ Transgender-T)	Marital status (Unmarried/ married)	Educa-tional status	Occu-pation	Monthly income (₹)	Dietary habits (Veg/ non-veg)	Addiction (Smoking Alcohol/ Drugs/ Others)	Health status (Healthy/ unhealthy)
1.										
2.										
3.										
4.										
5.										
6.										
7.										
8.										

Family Tree/Genogramme

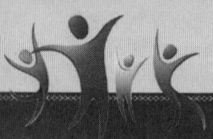

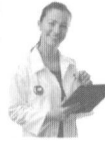

AVAILABILITY OF HEALTH CARE/SOCIAL/EDUCATIONAL FACILITIES

Facilities	Yes/No (If yes, specify name and distance from the house)
Nearby Health Care Facilities District hospital	
Government maternity hospital (if any)	
Private hospitals	
Subcenter	
Primary health center	
Community health center	
Indigenous medicine (hospital/clinic/dispensary)	
• Ayurveda	
• Yoga	
• Naturopathy	
• Unani	
• Siddha	
• Homeopathy	
• If other, specify	
Non-Governmental Organizations/Voluntary Health Organizations • Orphan age children	
• Physically challenged	
• Visually challenged	
• Mentally challenged	
• Hearing challenged	
• Women	
• Elderly	
• Youth welfare	
• Other	
Social Agencies • Post office	
• Bank	
• Police station	
Education Facilities **Government** • Anganwadis	
• Balwadis	
• Primary school	
• Elementary school	
• Secondary school	
• Senior secondary school	
• UG Institutions	
• PG institutions	
Private • Primary school	
• Elementary school	
• Secondary school	
• Senior secondary school	
• UG Institutions	
• PG institutions	

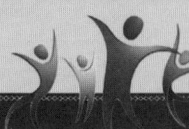
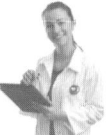

AVAILABILITY OF RECREATION/COMMUNICATION/TRANSPORT/RELIGIOUS FACILITIES

Facilities	Yes/No (If yes, specify name and distance from the house)
Recreation Facilities	
• Nearby market	
• Playgrounds	
• Public Gardens	
• Cinema halls	
• Clubs	
• Public library	
• Fairs	
• Festivals	
Communication Facilities	
• Telephone connection	
• Mobile phone	
• Internet facility	
• Letters	
Transport Facilities	
• Bus	
• Auto rickshaw	
• Taxi	
• Four wheeler	
• Two wheeler	
• Train	
• Airway	
Religious Places	
• Temple	
• Mosque	
• Gurudwara	
• Church	

Sketch of House

(Draw a sketch of the house showing location of rooms, doors, windows, entrance of the house, drinking water source, toilet and kitchen)

Key

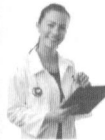

HOUSING STANDARDS AND ENVIRONMENTAL CONDITIONS

Characteristics	Parameters
Type of house	Pucca/Semi pucca/Katcha
Site	Elevated from surroundings/depressed from surroundings
Total number of living room	1/2/3/4/5/6/7/8/ _____
Space per person	Adequate (1 room -2 persons, 2 rooms -3 persons, 3 rooms – 5 persons, 4 rooms -7 persons, 5 or more rooms - 10 persons (additional 2 for each further room Inadequate (if above criteria is not fulfilled)
Ventilation	Adequate (doors and windows facing each other in each room) Inadequate (doors and windows not facing each other in each room)
Bathroom Hygiene	Not available/If available—Own/Public Hygienic/Unhygienic
Wall	Plastered or Cemented/Tiled/Wooden/Unplastered/Mud//Others, specify _____

Roof
  Height
  Painting
	
	Less than 10 feet/More than 10 feet
	Light colored/Dark colored

Day light	Adequate (Able to read the small fonts of newspaper inside the room during the day without any artificial lighting) Inadequate (Not able to read the small fonts of newspaper inside the room during the day without any artificial lighting)
Latrine Hygiene	Not available/If available—Own/Public Hygienic/Unhygienic
Electricity	Not available/Available
Drinking water supply	Tap/Well/Lake/Pond/Others, specify _____
Kitchen	Separate/Corner of the room/Others, specify _____
Type of fuel used	LPG/Electricity/Kerosene/Wood/Others, specify _____
Open space around the house	Absent/Present
Stagnant water around the house	Absent/Present
Street road	Tar/Cement/Mud/Others
Street light	Absent/Present

Modern sanitation facility
  Drainage system
  Sewage system
	
	Yes/No
	Yes/No

Drainage system	Closed/Open
Refuse disposal	Open dumping/Composting/Burning/Municipality collection/Community bins/Others, specify _____
Domestic animal	Absent/If present—Dog/Cow/Buffalo/Goat/Camel/Others, specify _____
Separate cattle shed (for the house with domestic animals)	Yes/No
Domestic birds/Poultry	Absent/If present—Hen/Cock/Parrot/Others, specify _____
Separate poultry shed/cage (for the house with domestic birds)	Yes/No
Rodents	Absent/If present—Rat/Others, specify _____
Street animals	Absent/If present—Dogs/Cats/Cows/Others, specify _____
Insect vectors	Absent/If present—Mosquitoes/Flies/Ticks/Others, specify _____

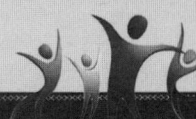

SOCIOECONOMIC STATUS

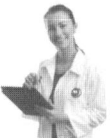

Social class/Socioeconomic status (according to rural/urban socioeconomic scale, Refer to Annexures)

_____

VULNERABLE/TARGET GROUPS IN THE FAMILY

Total eligible couples _____   Children (0–1 years) _____   Adolescent Girls _____

Total postnatal mothers _____   Children (1–3 years) _____   Elderly (above 60 years) _____

Total antenatal mothers _____   Children (3–5 years) _____   Other, specify _____

MONTHLY FAMILY BUDGET

	Income			Expenditure	
Sources	**Income (In ₹)**	**Income (In Percentage)**	**Sources**	**Expenditure (In ₹)**	**Expenditure (In Percentage)**
Salary			House rent		
Rent			Education		
Agriculture			Food		
Animals			Fuel (LPG)		
Pension			Fuel (Petrol/Diesel)		
Stipend			Clothing		
Part time business			Entertainment		
Others			Electricity		
			Water		
			Property taxes		
			Telephone/Internet		
			Transportation		
			Health		
			Festival		
			Saving		
			Insurance		
			Others		
Total (₹)			**Total (₹)**		

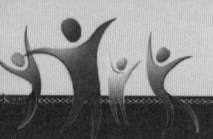
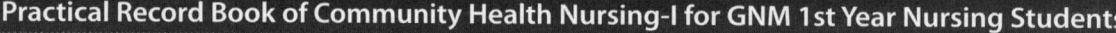
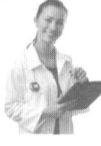

FAMILY DIETARY PATTERN

Food groups	Food items	Food consumption (Yes/No)	Frequency of consumption (Servings per day or per week)	Method/Form of food preparation (Boiling/steaming/raw/ pressure cooking/ frying/germination, etc.)	Method of food storage at home (Hygienic-H/ Unhygienic-U)
Energy giving foods	Rice				
	Wheat				
	Tubers				
	Edible oil				
	Ghee				
	Butter				
Body building foods	Meat				
	Fish				
	Poultry				
	Eggs				
	Pulses				
Protective foods	Vegetables				
	Fruits				
	Milk & milk products				
Beverages	Tea				
	Coffee				
	Water				
Others	Junk food				

SOCIOCULTURAL ASPECTS

Menstruation _____

_____

_____

_____

_____

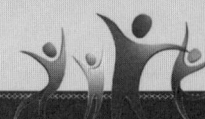
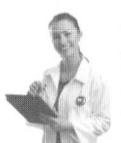

Antenatal Care _____
_____
_____
_____
_____
_____

Child Birth _____
_____
_____
_____
_____
_____

Postnatal Care _____
_____
_____
_____
_____
_____

Care of Sick _____
_____
_____
_____
_____
_____
_____

Food Consumption _____
_____
_____
_____
_____
_____
_____

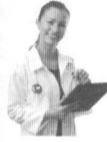

FAMILY PLANNING STATUS (ELIGIBLE COUPLE)

S. No.	Name of the eligible couple (Mr. _____ Mrs _____)	Age (yrs.)/ Sex (Male-M Female-F)	Family planning practice (a) Yes (b) No	Temporary family planning method					Permanent family planning method		Month and year of adoption/ Duration of use
				Condom	Oral pills	Copper-T	Inject able	Implant	Tubectomy	Vasectomy	
1.											
2.											
3.											
4.											

IMMUNIZATION STATUS

Age Group	Weeks/ Months/Years	Current Vaccine Under UIP (2017)	Child Name/Vaccines/Date of Administration (DOA)					
			Child -1 _____		Child -2 _____		Child -3 _____	
			Vaccines	DOA	Vaccines	DOA	Vaccines	DOA
Infant	At birth	BCG, OPV-0, Hep-B birth dose						
	6 weeks	OPV-1, Rota-1, Pentavalent-1, IPV-1, PCV-1						
	10 weeks	OPV-2, Rota-2, Pentavalent-2						
	14 weeks	OPV-3, Rota-3, Pentavalent-3, IPV-2, PCV-2						
	9 months	MR/Measles-1, Vit-A*, JE-1#, PCV-Booster						
Under five children	16–24 months	DPT-Booster-1, OPV-Booster, MR/Measles-2, JE-2#						
School going	5–6 Years	DPT-Booster -2						
Adolescent	10 years	TT-1						
	16 years	TT-2						
Pregnancy		TT-1						
		TT-2						

*Vitamin A to be given every 6 months till five years of age and a separate chart is given below for documentation. #JE vaccine given in selected districts. **BCG:** Bacillus Calmette-Guerin; **Pentavalent [DPT:** diphtheria-pertussis-tetanus; **Hep B:** Hepatitis B; **Hib:** Haemophilus influenzae type b]; **JE:** Japanese Encephalitis; **MR/Measles/MMR:** Measles Mumps rubella; **OPV:** oral polio vaccine; **TT:** tetanus toxoid; **IPV:** inactivated poliovirus vaccine. **Rota-** Rotavirus vaccine, **PCV:** Pneumonia; Additional _____

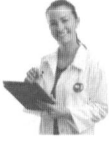

Age (in months) →		9	18	24	30	36	42	48	54	60
Dose →		1st	2nd	3rd	4th	5th	6th	7th	8th	9th
Vitamin-A Solution (DOA)	Child-1 _____									
	Child-2 _____									
	Child-3 _____									

VITAL EVENTS IN THE FAMILY DURING THE LAST ONE YEAR

Birth (if any)

S. No.	Name	Date of birth	Sex	Parents name	Place of Birth	Birth Registration- Yes/No
1.						
2.						
3.						

Death (if any)

S. No.	Name	Date of death	Age/ Sex	Cause of death	Place of death	Death Registration- Yes/No
1.						
2.						
3.						

Marriage (if any)

S. No.	Name of the Couple	Age		Date of marriage	Marriage Registration- Yes/No
		Wife	Husband		
1.					
2.					
3.					

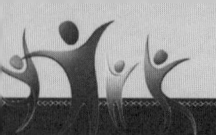
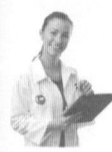

Family Health Profile

Instructions

1. Select a key case(s) from the assigned family—elderly/adult/adolescent/antenatal/postnatal/newborn/under five/physically challenged/sick/vulnerable or specific group as per assigned family priority health need.

2. Write the selected family member(s)—identification data, health history, specific physical assessment, lab investigations (if any), medications, diet chart, identified health needs/problems and disease condition (book picture)

3. Eight blank pages are provided here. If more details are required, paste the additional pages in the record book.

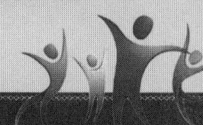
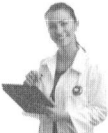

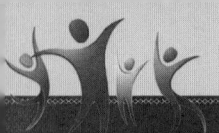

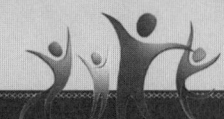

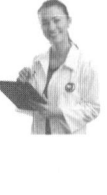

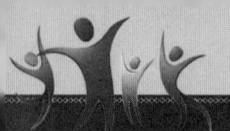

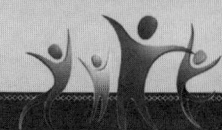

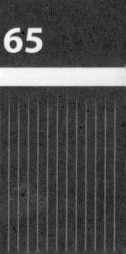

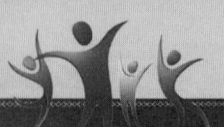

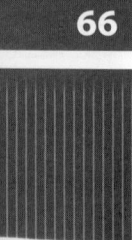

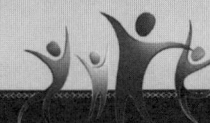
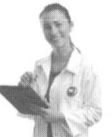

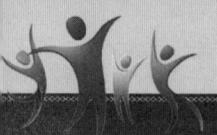

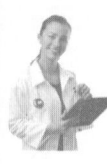

Instructions
1. Identify the family health needs, prioritize them, formulate the possible nursing diagnosis and write the nursing care plan.
2. If more details are required, paste the additional pages in the record book.

Identified Health Problems/Needs

_____
_____
_____
_____
_____
_____

Prioritization of Health Problems/Needs

_____
_____
_____
_____
_____
_____

Priority Nursing Diagnosis

_____
_____
_____
_____
_____
_____
_____
_____
_____
_____
_____

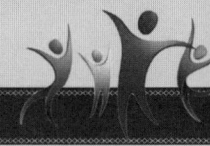

FAMILY HEALTH NURSING CARE PLAN

Assessment	Diagnosis	Goal/ Objective	Planning	Implementation	Evaluation

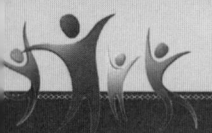

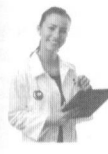

FAMILY HEALTH NURSING CARE PLAN

Assessment	Diagnosis	Goal/Objective	Planning	Implementation	Evaluation

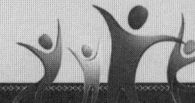

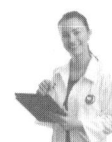

FAMILY HEALTH NURSING CARE PLAN

Assessment	Diagnosis	Goal/ Objective	Planning	Implementation	Evaluation

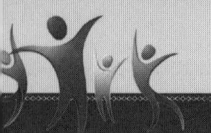
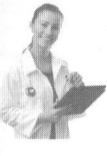

FAMILY HEALTH NURSING CARE PLAN

Assessment	Diagnosis	Goal/Objective	Planning	Implementation	Evaluation

HEALTH EDUCATION

REFERENCES

Signature of Student

Signature of Supervisor

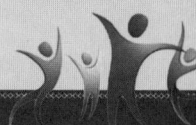

3. Health Assessment

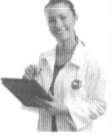

3.1. Adult

IDENTIFICATION DATA

Name: _____

Address: _____

Age/Sex: _____

Religion—Hindu/Muslims/Sikh/Christian/Others: _____

Caste—GEN/SC/ST/OBC: _____

Marital Status—Unmarried/Married: _____

Occupation—Unemployed/Government/Private Job/Self-Employed/Daily Wage Worker/Homemaker/Others: _____

_____

Language Known—Hindi/English/Others: _____

Relation with Head of the Family: _____

Family Size (Total Members): _____

Family Type—Nuclear/Joint: _____

Monthly Family Income ₹:_____

Family Income per Capita ₹: _____

Nearby Sub-center/PHC/CHC/District Hospital: _____

Classification/Diagnosis: _____

BRIEF HISTORY

History of Present Complaints

(Character/onset/location/duration/severity pattern/associated factors/medication and treatment) _____

_____

_____

_____

_____

Past Health (Medical/Surgical) History

(Problems at birth/infancy/childhood/immunization/adulthood (physical, mental, and psychological)/allergies (food/medication/others)/Chronic illness (e.g. hypertension, diabetes mellitus, heart, liver, renal disease etc./hereditary/communicable disease/any surgery and reason/other history) _____

_____

_____

_____

_____

_____

_____

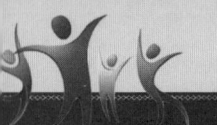

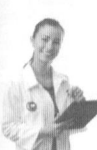

Menstrual History

Age at menarche: _____ years   **Menstruation:** Regular/irregular   **Length of cycle:** _____ days

Duration of blood flow: _____ days   LMP _____   Age at Menopause _____ year

Dysmenorrhea: Present/Absent   **Leucorrhea:** Present/Absent   **Menorrhagia:** Present/Absent

Marital History

Age at marriage _____ years   Duration of marriage _____ years

Consanguineous marriage—Yes/No   Relationship with spouse—satisfactory/unsatisfactory

Obstetric History

S. No	Year	Pregnancy (normal/ complicated)	Type of delivery (Normal/Assisted/LSCS)	Place of Delivery (Hospital/ Home)	Delivery conducted by (Doctor/Nurse/ Dai/Other)	Alive/ still borne	Sex	Birth-weight (in kg)	Present condition (Alive/ dead)
1.									
2.									
3.									
4.									
5.									
6.									

Personal and Social History

Dietary pattern (veg/non-veg/lacto-ovo-vegetarian)/No. of meals per day/staple food/fasting habits

_____

_____

_____

_____

_____

Bowel and bladder habit (regular/irregular, stool frequency and consistency)

_____

_____

_____

_____

_____

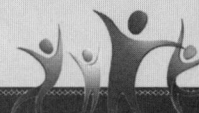

Rest/sleep/activity/exercise/travel

_____
_____
_____

Occupation (Type/working hours per day/work place stress/job satisfaction)

_____
_____
_____
_____

Habits (Alcohol/smoking/drugs/tobacco/chewing betel leaves)

_____
_____
_____
_____

Leisure/recreational/religious/spiritual activities

_____
_____
_____
_____

Relationship with family members/relatives/friends/others—satisfactory/unsatisfactory

_____
_____
_____
_____

FAMILY COMPOSITION AND CHARACTERISTICS

S. No.	Name of the family members	Relationship with head of the family	Date of birth/ sex (Male-M/ Female-F/ Transgender-T)	Marital status (Unmarried/ Married)	Educa-tional status	Occu-pation	Monthly income (₹)	Dietary habits (Veg/ Non-veg)	Addiction (Smoking Alcohol/ Drugs/ Others)	Health status (Healthy/ Unhealthy)
1.										
2.										
3.										
4.										
5.										
6.										
7.										
8.										

Family Tree/Genogramme

Key

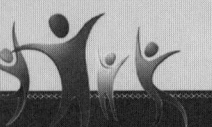
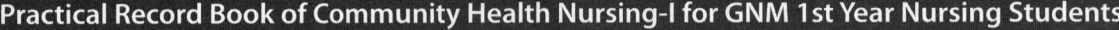
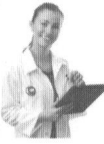

HOUSING STANDARDS AND ENVIRONMENTAL CONDITIONS

Characteristics	Parameters
Type of house	Pucca/Semi-pucca/Katcha
Total number of living room	1/2/3/4/5/6/7/8/ _____
Ventilation	Adequate (Doors and windows facing each other in each room) Inadequate (Doors and windows not facing each other in each room)
Bathroom	Not available/If available—Own/Public
Latrine	Not available/If available—Own/Public
Electricity	Not available/Available
Drinking water supply	Tap/Well/Lake/Pond/Others, specify _____
Kitchen	Separate/Corner of the room/Others, specify_____
Type of fuel used	LPG/Electricity/Kerosene/Wood/Others, specify _____

Modern sanitation facility
   Drainage system
   Sewage system
	
	 Yes/No
	 Yes/No

Drainage system	Closed/Open
Refuse disposal	Open dumping/Composting/Burning/Municipality collection/Community bins/Others, specify _____
Domestic animal	Not present/If present—Dog/Cow/Buffalo/Goat/Camel/Others, specify _____
Separate cattle shed (for the house with domestic animals)	Yes/No
Rodents	Not present/If yes—Rat/Others, specify _____
Street animals	Not present/If yes—Dogs/Cats/Cows/Others, specify _____
Insect vectors	Not present/If yes—Mosquitoes/Flies/Ticks/Others, specify _____

Recreation facilities: Market/playgrounds/cinema halls/clubs/public library/fairs

Communication facilities: Telephone connection/mobile phone/internet facility/letters

Transport facilities: Bus/auto rickshaw/taxi/four wheeler/two wheeler/train/airway

Religious places: Temple/Mosque/Gurudwara/Church

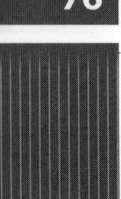

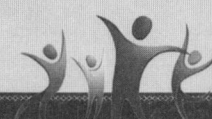
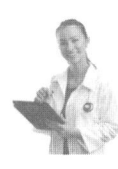

PHYSICAL EXAMINATION (put a tick (✓) mark wherever necessary or mention the finding in the provided space if needed)

General Appearance

Consciousness: Conscious/semiconscious/unconscious/confused
Posture: Normal/kyphosis/lordosis/scoliosis
Body built: Thin/moderate/obese
Nourishment: Well-nourished/under nourished
Activity: Active/dull/lethargic
Dress/grooming: Well-groomed/dirty
Gait (ability to walk/move): Normal/unsteady/any limp
Look: Normal/anxious/depressed/fear

Anthropometric Measurement

Weight: _____kg, Height: _____ cm, BMI (Quetelet's Index)_____[weight (kg)/height^2(meter)]
Waist circumference _____cm
Hip circumference _____cm
Waist/Hip Ratio- _____ (normal < 0.85)

Vital Signs

Temperature _____°C, Pulse_____beats/m,
Respiration _____breaths/m, BP _____ mm Hg,
Pain (5th vital sign)-absent/if present-onset/intensity/duration/type/location
_____
_____
_____

Skin Condition

Color: Normal/redness/flushing/cyanosis/jaundice/ pallor/pigmented/white patches
Texture: Smooth/soft/rough/dry/wrinkled/edematous
Lesions: Absent/macule/papule/vesicle/pustule/ulcer/scab
Temperature: Normal (warm)/cool/hot
Turgor (elasticity): Normal/decreased
_____

Head

Shape: Symmetrical/asymmetrical
Scalp: Normal/lesion/lump/infection/psoriasis
Hair: Color: Normal/gray/white/artificial color
     Texture: Smooth/rough/dry/flaky/oily/thin
     Dandruff: Present/absent
     Alopecia: Present/absent
     Pediculosis: Present/absent
     Hygiene: Good/poor

Face

Shape: Symmetrical/asymmetrical
Color: Normal/pale/flushed
Edema: Present/absent
Movement: Normal/tics/tremors/fasciculation
_____
_____

Eyes

Eye	Right	Left
Discharge: Present/absent		
Eyebrows: Symmetrical/asymmetrical/absent		
Eyelids: Normal/edema/ptosis/entropion/ectropion		
Eyelashes: Normal/stye/infection		
Eyeball: Normal/protruded/sunken		
Sclera: Normal/jaundice/redness		
Conjunctiva: Normal/moist/pale/red/watery/purulent		
Pupils: Cloudy/dilated/constricted/reacting to light		
Vision: Normal/myopia/hyperopia		
Glasses/contact lens: Present/absent		

Ears

Ear	Right	Left
Shape: Symmetrical/asymmetrical with head		
External ear: Normal/discharge/ear wax accumulation/pain/itching		
Auditory canal: Smooth/pink/redness/discharge/wax plug/lesion/foreign body		
Tympanic membrane: Intact/redness/swelling/perforated/bulging		
Gross hearing: Normal/using hearing aid		

Nose

Discharge/crust: Present/absent
Nasal septum: Intact/perforated/deviation _____
Mucous membrane: Normal (moist & red)/dry/lesion/discharge/swollen/epistaxis
Polyp: Present/absent
Flaring: Present/absent

Mouth

Odor: Normal/foul smelling
Lips: Normal (pink, moist, smooth)/dry/cracked/cyanosis/swelling/redness/crust/cheilosis
Gums: Normal (pink and smooth)/swelling/bleeding/pus/gingivitis
Tongue/mucus: Normal (pink and moist)/pale/dry/coated/redness/lesion/swelling/glossitis
Teeth: Normal/poor alignment/missing/dental caries/plaque/discoloration _____
Tonsils: Normal (small, pink, symmetrical)/inflammation/enlarged/lesion/exudate
Throat and pharynx: Normal/redness/pus/lesion/exudate

77

contd…

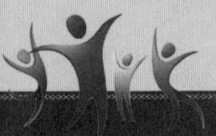

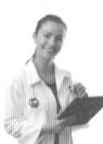

Neck

Lymph nodes (preauricular, parotid, postauricular, occipital, tonsillar, submaxillary, submental, anterior and deep cervical chain, posterior cervical, supraclavicular)- non-palpable/enlarge/tender

Thyroid gland: Normal (soft and elastic)/asymmetrical/enlarge/lump/bulging

Range of motion (flexion/extension/rotation): Symmetrical/asymmetrical neck with ROM

Chest

Shape/contour: Symmetrical/asymmetrical

Breathing pattern: Normal/unequal chest expansion/use of accessory muscles

Breath sounds: Normal/abnormal-wheezing/rhonchi/crackles/stridor/others _____

Sputum: Absent/if present, color/consistency _____

Heart rate: Normal/fast/slow _____

Heart rhythm: Regular/irregular _____

Heart sounds: Normal/abnormal-murmur/others _____

Female Breast

Breast	Right	Left
Size: Round/smooth/retraction/dimpling/lump/swollen/tender Shape: Symmetrical/asymmetrical		
Areola: Normal(moist, round)/dry Nipple: Everted/inversion/flat/cracked/crusted/discharge Axillary lymph nodes: Non-palpable/mobile/enlarge/tender Mass or lump: Absent/location/shape/size/consistency/tenderness		

Monthly Breast Self-Examination: Yes/No

Abdomen

Inspection

Shape: Symmetrical/asymmetrical/distension/observable mass/hernia/ascites/unusual pulsation

Color: Normal/white and silver lines (striae)

Skin: Normal/lesion/rashes/previous surgery scar/vascularity

Auscultation

Bowel sounds: Present/absent/frequency _____ movements/min

Palpation

Superficial palpation: Soft/pain/tenderness/mass _____

Deep palpation (in all 4 quadrants for palpable organs): No organomegaly/pain/tenderness/palpable- liver/spleen/urinary bladder/appendix/inguinal hernia _____

Percussion: Presence of gas/fluid/mass (dullness)/liver margins _____

Extremities

Upper extremities: Right Left	Right	Left
Range of motion: Symmetrical/asymmetrical Fingers: Normal/polydactyly/syndactyly arachnodactyly/edema/tremors/nodules/crepitus/pain Nails Color: Pink/pale/cyanosis Shape: Normal (convex)/spoon-shaped/beau's lines/flat/clubbed Hygiene: Clean/dirty/long/short		

Capillary refill time.......seconds (Normal <3 seconds)

Lower Extremities	Right	Left
Range of motion: Symmetrical/asymmetrical Toe/foot: Normal/polydactyly/syndactyly/arachnodactyly/nodule/edema/pain/alignment/position/shape _____ Joint: Normal/warm/swollen/tender/painful Nails: Color: Pink/pale/cyanosis Shape: Normal (convex)/spoon-shaped/beau's lines/flat/clubbed Hygiene: Clean/dirty/long/short Varicose veins: Present/absent		

Rectum

Rectum and anus: Normal/hemorrhoids/fissures/polyp/ulcer/lesion/rashes/redness/bleeding

Stool: Color/odor/consistency _____

Sacrococcygeal area: Swelling/redness/dimpling or hair

Bowel pattern: Regular/irregular

Urinary Bladder

Bladder pattern: Normal/burning micturition/dribbling of urine while working or coughing

Urine: Color/odor/frequency _____

contd…

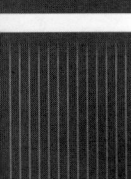

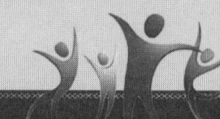
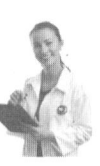

Genitals	Male genitalia
Female Genitalia	Scrotum: Symmetrical/asymmetrical/lesions/redness/swelling/pain/discharge/mass _____
Mons pubis: Normal/lesions/redness/edema	_____
Labia majora: Normal/lesions/redness/edema	Penis: Normal/tenderness/pain/discharge
Perineum: Normal/lesions/redness/edema	Foreskin: Intact/retractable/lesions
Vagina: Normal/redness/lesion/discharge/pain _____	Location of urinary orifice: Normal/ventral/dorsal surface
Urethra: Normal/discharge/redness/swelling _____	Urethra: Normal/discharge/redness/swelling
Inguinal lymph nodes: Normal/enlarge/tender/palpable	Inguinal lymph nodes: Normal/enlarge/tender/palpable
	Inguinal hernia: Absent/present
	Monthly Testicular Self-Examination: Yes/No

LAB INVESTIGATIONS

S. No.	Date/time	Investigation	Patient value	Normal value	Remarks

MEDICATIONS

S. No.	Name and action	Dose/route/frequency	Indication	Side effects

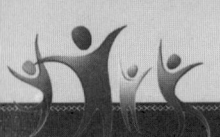

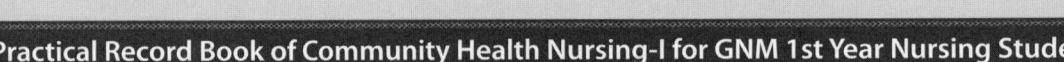

DIET CHART

_____

_____

_____

_____

_____

_____

_____

_____

_____

_____

_____

_____

_____

_____

_____

_____

_____

_____

_____

_____

_____

_____

_____

_____

_____

_____

_____

_____

_____

_____

_____

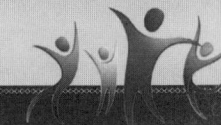

Identified Health Problems/Needs

_____

_____

_____

_____

_____

_____

_____

_____

_____

Prioritization of Health Problems/Needs

_____

_____

_____

_____

_____

_____

_____

_____

_____

Priority Nursing Diagnosis

_____

_____

_____

_____

_____

_____

_____

_____

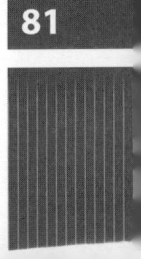

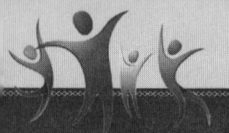

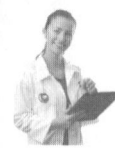

NURSING CARE PLAN

Assessment	Diagnosis	Goal/ Objective	Planning	Implementation	Evaluation

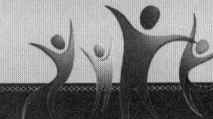

NURSING CARE PLAN

Assessment	Diagnosis	Goal/ Objective	Planning	Implementation	Evaluation

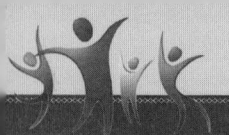

HEALTH EDUCATION

(Include diet/medication and its side effects/exercise/rest/self-care/hygiene/follow-up)

_____
_____
_____
_____
_____
_____
_____
_____
_____
_____
_____
_____
_____
_____
_____
_____
_____
_____
_____

REFERENCES

_____
_____
_____
_____
_____
_____

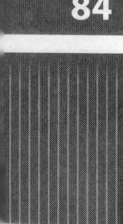

Signature of Student   **Signature of Supervisor**

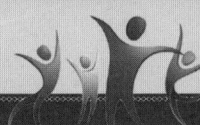

3.2. Elderly

IDENTIFICATION DATA

Name: _____

Address: _____

Age/Sex: _____

Religion—Hindu/Muslims/Sikh/Christian/Others: _____

Caste—GEN/SC/ST/OBC: _____

Marital Status—Unmarried/Married: _____

Occupation—Unemployed/Government/Private Job/Self-Employed/Daily Wage Worker/Homemaker/Others: _____
_____

Language Known—Hindi/English/Others: _____

Relation with Head of the Family: _____

Family Size (Total Members): _____

Family Type—Nuclear/Joint: _____

Monthly Family Income ₹: _____

Family Income per Capita ₹: _____

Nearby Sub-center/PHC/CHC/District Hospital: _____

Classification/Diagnosis: _____

Brief History

History of present complaints (character/onset/location/duration/severity pattern/associated factors/medication and treatment)

_____

_____

_____

_____

_____

_____

Past health (medical/surgical) history (problems at birth/infancy/childhood/immunization/adulthood (physical, mental, and psychological)/allergies (food/medication/others)/Chronic illness (e.g. hypertension, diabetes mellitus, heart, liver, renal disease etc./hereditary/communicable disease/any surgery and reason/other history)

_____

_____

_____

_____

_____

_____

_____

_____

_____

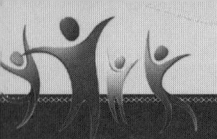

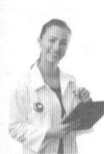

Menstrual History

Age at menarche: _____ years   **Menstruation:** Regular/irregular   **Length of cycle:**_____ days
Duration of blood flow: _____ days   **Dysmenorrhea:** Present/Absent _____   **Leucorrhea:** Present/Absent_____
Menorrhagia: Present/Absent   Age at Menopause_____ year   **Postmenstrual bleeding:** Present/Absent _____

Marital History

Age at marriage _____ years   Duration of marriage _____ years   **Consanguineous marriage:** Yes/No
Relationship with spouse: Satisfactory/unsatisfactory   **Sexual activity:** Active/Inactive

Obstetric History

S. No	Year	Pregnancy (normal/complicated)	Type of delivery (Normal/Assisted/LSCS)	Place of delivery (Hospital/Home)	Delivery conducted by (Doctor/Nurse/Dai/Other)	Alive/still borne	Sex	Birth-weight (in kg)	Present condition (Alive/dead)
1.									
2.									
3.									
4.									
5.									
6.									

Personal and Social History

Dietary pattern (Veg/non-veg/lacto-ovo-vegetarian)/No. of meals per day/food choices/availability of food/related health problems

_____

_____

_____

Bowel and bladder habit (regular/irregular, stool-frequency and consistency)

_____

_____

Rest/sleep/activity/exercise/travel

_____

_____

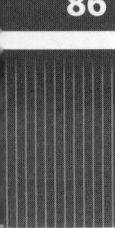

Occupation (Past and present occupation/duration of employment and retirement/pension plan/other sources of income/part-time job)

_____

_____

_____

Habits (Alcohol/smoking/drugs/tobacco/chewing betel leaves)

_____

_____

_____

Leisure/hobbies/recreational/religious/spiritual activities

_____

_____

_____

Relationship with family members, relatives, friends, others/status of elderly in the family/family support in elderly care/elder abuse

_____

_____

_____

If living alone—its reason/surviving family members/support from relatives, friends, neighbors, periodicity of contact with them/pets

_____

_____

_____

Assess to telephone/mobile/internet/emergency contact no. (family member/friends/relatives/doctor/police etc.)

_____

_____

_____

FAMILY COMPOSITION AND CHARACTERISTICS

S. No.	Name of the family members	Relationship with head of the family	Date of birth/ sex (Male-M/ Female-F/ Transgender-T)	Marital status (Unmarried/ Married)	Educa- tional status	Occu- pation	Monthly income (₹)	Dietary habits (Veg/ Non-veg)	Addiction (Smoking Alcohol/ Drugs/ Others)	Health status (Healthy/ Unhealthy)
1.										
2.										
3.										
4.										
5.										
6.										
7.										
8.										

Family Tree/Genogramme

Key

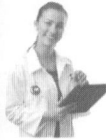

HOUSING STANDARDS AND ENVIRONMENTAL CONDITIONS

Characteristics	Parameters
Type of house	Pucca/Semi-pucca/Katcha
Total number of living room	1/2/3/4/5/6/7/8/ _____
Ventilation	Adequate (Doors and windows facing each other in each room) Inadequate (Doors and windows not facing each other in each room)
Bathroom	Not available/If available—Own/Public
Latrine	Not available/If available—Own/Public
Electricity	Not available/Available
Drinking water supply	Tap/Well/Lake/Pond/Others, specify _____
Kitchen	Separate/Corner of the room/Others, specify _____
Type of fuel used	LPG/Electricity/Kerosene/Wood/Others, specify _____

Modern sanitation facility
   Drainage system
   Sewage system
	
	Yes/No
	Yes/No

Drainage system	Closed/Open
Refuse disposal	Open dumping/Composting/Burning/Municipality collection/Community bins/Others, specify _____
Domestic animal	Not present/If present—Dog/Cow/Buffalo/Goat/Camel/Others, specify _____
Separate cattle shed (for the house with domestic animals)	Yes/No
Rodents	Not present/If yes—Rat/Others, specify _____
Street animals	Not present/If yes—Dogs/Cats/Cows/Others, specify _____
Insect vectors	Not present/If yes—Mosquitoes/Flies/Ticks/Others, specify _____

Recreation facilities: Market/playgrounds/cinema halls/clubs/public library/fairs

Communication facilities: Telephone connection/mobile phone/internet facility/letters

Transport facilities: Bus/auto rickshaw/taxi/four wheeler/two wheeler/train/airway

Religious places: Temple/Mosque/Gurudwara/Church

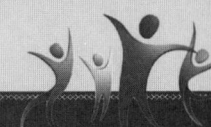
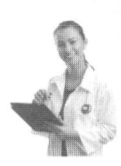

PHYSICAL EXAMINATION (put a tick (✓) mark wherever necessary or mention the finding in the provided space if needed)

General Appearance

Consciousness- conscious/semiconscious/unconscious/confused
Posture: Normal/kyphosis/lordosis/scoliosis
Body built: Thin/moderate/obese
Nourishment: Well-nourished/under nourished
Activity: Active/dull/lethargic
Dress/grooming: Well-groomed/dirty
Gait (ability to walk/move)- normal/unsteady/any limp
Look: Normal/anxious/depressed/fear

Anthropometric Measurement

Weight _____kg, Height _____ cm, BMI (Quetelet's Index)_____ [weight (kg)/height^2(meter)]
Waist circumference _____ cm
Hip circumference _____ cm
Abdominal fat Accumulation-Yes/No_____(if Waist/Hip Ratio- < 0.85)

Vital Signs

Temperature -_____°C, Pulse- _____beats/m,
Respiration _____ breaths/m,
BP _____ mm of Hg, (high/low)
Pain (5th vital sign)-onset/intensity/duration/type/location
_____
_____

Skin Condition

Color: Normal/pigmented/age spots/redness/flushing/cyanosis/jaundice/pallor/white patches
Texture: Smooth/soft/wrinkled/loose/scaling/sagging/rough/dry/oily/edematous
Eruptions: Absent/present _____
Itching: Absent/present
Masses: Absent/present _____
Unhealed or irregular sore/mole: Absent/present
Temperature: Normal (warm)/cool/hot
Bed sore: Present/absent

Head

Shape: Symmetrical/asymmetrical
Scalp: Normal/lesion/lump/infection/psoriasis
Hair: Color: Normal/gray/white/artificial color
　　　Texture: Smooth/rough/dry/flaky/oily/thin
　　　Dandruff: Present/absent
　　　Alopecia: Present/absent
　　　Pediculosis: Present/absent
　　　Hygiene: Good/poor

Face

Shape: Symmetrical/asymmetrical
Color: Normal/pale/flushed
Edema: Present/absent
Hirsutism: Present/absent

Eyes

Eye	Right	Left
Discharge: Present/absent		
Eyelids: Normal/edema/ptosis/entropion/ectropion		
Eyelashes: Normal/stye/infection		
Eyeball: Normal/protruded/sunken		
Sclera: Normal/slight yellowish/jaundice/redness		
Conjunctiva: Normal/moist/pale/red/watery/purulent		
Pupils: Cloudy/dilated/constricted/reacting to light		
Tearing: Present/absent		
Vision: Normal/myopia/hyperopia/blurred/glaucoma/cataract		
Glasses/contact lens: Present/absent		

Ears

Ear	Right	Left
External ear: Normal/discharge/ear wax accumulation/pain/itching		
Auditory canal: Smooth/pink/redness/discharge/wax plug/lesion/foreign body		
Tympanic membrane: Intact/redness/swelling/perforated/bulging		
Gross hearing: Normal/difficulty in hearing/tinnitus/using hearing aid		

Nose

Discharge/crust: Present/absent
Nasal septum: Intact/perforated/deviation _____
Mucous membrane: Normal (moist & red)/dry/lesion/discharge/swollen/epistaxis
Polyp: Present/absent
Sense of smell: Normal decreased

Mouth

Odor: Normal/foul smelling
Lips: Normal (pink, moist, smooth)/dry/cracked/cyanosis/swelling/redness/crust/cheilosis
Gums: Normal (pink and smooth)/swelling/bleeding/pus/gingivitis
Tongue/mucus: Normal (pink and moist)/pale/dry/coated/fissures/redness/lesion/swelling/glossitis
Teeth: Normal/missing/dentures/loose/dental caries/plaque/discoloration _____

contd…

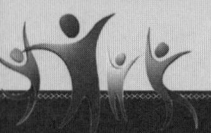
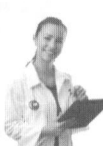

Appetite: Normal/decreased

Sense of taste: Normal/altered

Chewing: Normal/difficult

Swallowing: Normal/difficult

Dry Mouth: Present/absent

Any devices: No/feeding tubes/parenteral nutrition/ostomy

Throat and pharynx: Normal/redness/pus/lesion/exudates

Monthly Oral Self-Examination: Yes/no

Neck

Lymph nodes (preauricular, parotid, postauricular, occipital, tonsillar, submaxillary, submental, anterior and deep cervical chain, posterior cervical, supraclavicular)- non-palpable/enlarge/tender

Thyroid gland: Normal (soft and elastic)/asymmetrical/enlarge/lump/bulging

Neck movement: Normal/pain/stiffness

Chest

Shape/contour: Symmetrical/asymmetrical

Breathing pattern: Normal/dyspnea/excessive sneezing/excessive coughing/unequal chest expansion/pain in exertion/palpitation in exertion/shortness of breath

Breath sounds: Normal/abnormal-wheezing/rhonchi/crackles/stridor/others _____

Sputum: Absent/if present, color/consistency _____
_____

Heart rate: Normal/fast/slow _____

Heart rhythm: Regular/irregular _____

Heart sounds: Normal/abnormal-murmur/others _____

Blood Pressure: Normal/decreased/increased

Exercise intolerance: Present/absent

Female Breast

Breast	Right	Left
Size: Round/pendulous/retraction/dimpling/lump/tender Shape: Symmetrical/asymmetrical Areola: Normal(moist, round)/dry Nipple: Normal/everted/inversion/flat/cracked/crusted/any discharge _____		
Axillary lymph nodes: Non-palpable/mobile/enlarge/tender Mass or lump: Absent/if present, location/shape/size/consistency/tenderness _____		

Monthly Breast Self-Examination: Yes/No

Abdomen

Inspection

Shape: Symmetrical/asymmetrical/distension/observable mass/hernia/ascites/unusual pulsation

Color: Normal/white and silver lines (striae)

Skin: Normal/lesion/rashes/previous surgery scar/vascularity

Auscultation

Bowel sounds: Present/absent/frequency ____ movements/min

Palpation

Superficial palpation: Soft/pain/tenderness/mass _____
_____

Deep palpation (in all 4 quadrants for palpable organs) – no organomegaly/pain/tenderness/palpable- liver/spleen/urinary bladder/appendix/inguinal hernia _____

Percussion: Presence of gas/fluid/mass (dullness)/liver margins
_____

Digestion: Normal/sluggish/heart burn/belching/distension

Extremities

Upper extremities	Right	Left
Range of motion: Symmetrical/asymmetrical/decreased		
Fingers: Normal/polydactylyl/syndactyl/rachnodactyl/edema/tremors (shaking)/nodules/crepitus/pain		
Joint: Normal/stiffness/warm/swollen/tender/painful		
Nails: Color-pink/pale/cyanosis		
Shape/texture: Normal (convex)/spoon-shaped/beau's lines/flat/clubbed/thick/brittle		
Nail hygiene: Clean/dirty/long/short		

Capillary refill time _____ seconds (Normal <3 seconds)

Lower extremities	Right	Left
Range of motion-symmetrical/asymmetrical/decreased Toe/foot: Normal/polydactyly/syndactyly/arachnodactyly/nodule/edema/pain/alignment/position/shape _____		
Joint: Normal/stiffness/warm/swollen /tender/painful		
Nails: Color-pink/pale/cyanosis		
Shape/texture: Normal (convex)/spoon-shaped/beau's lines/flat/clubbed/thick/brittle		
Use of walking aid: No/If yes—stick/crutches/prosthesis		
Hygiene: Clean/dirty/long/short		
Varicose veins: Present/absent		

Rectum

Rectum and anus: Normal/hemorrhoids/fissures/polyp/ulcer/lesion/rashes/redness/bleeding

Stool: Color/odor/consistency _____
_____

Bowel pattern: Regular/irregular

Defecation: Normal/painful/bleeding/diarrhea/constipation

90

contd…

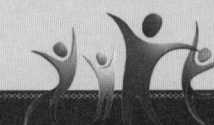
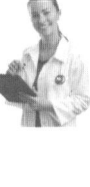

Urinary Bladder

Bladder pattern: Normal/dysuria/nocturia/hematuria/polyuria/burning micturition/dribbling of urine while working or coughing/incontinence

Urine: Color/odor/frequency _____
_____

Genitals

Female Genitalia

Vagina: Normal/itching/dry/pain/redness/lesion/discharge

Urethra: Normal/discharge/redness/swelling _____

Inguinal lymph nodes: Normal/enlarge/tender/palpable

Male Genitalia

Scrotum: Normal/pendulous/symmetrical/asymmetrical/lesions/redness/swelling/pain/discharge/mass _____

Penis: Normal/tenderness/pain/discharge/lesions

Urethra: Normal/discharge/redness/swelling

Inguinal lymph nodes: Normal/enlarge/tender/palpable

Inguinal hernia: Absent/present

Monthly Testicular Self-Examination: Yes/No

Neurological Assessment

Coordination and balance: Normal/decrease/abnormal

Pain perception: Normal/decrease/absent

Touch perception: Normal/decrease/absent

Hot perception: Normal/decrease/absent

Cold perception: Normal/decrease/absent

Headache/seizures: Absent/present

Syncope/fainting attacks: Absent/present

Dizziness: Absent/present

Giddiness: Absent/present

Numbness in hand or feet: Absent/present

Tremors: Absent/present

Dementia/Forgetfulness

Recall 3 items at 1 minute: <2 items/2 items/all 3 items

Name as many as animals as in 1 minutes—normal (able to recall 18 or more animals in 1 minute)/abnormal (able to recall less than 12 animals in 1 minute)

ACTIVITIES OF DAILY LIVING (ADL)

S. No.	Daily living activities	°	Yes/No
	Personal tasks		
1.	Eat food by self		
2.	Drink fluids by self		
3.	Go to toilet by self		
4.	Able to control bladder		
5.	Able to control bowel		
6.	Go to bathroom by self		
7.	Bath by self		
8.	Dress and undress by self		
9.	Cut or clean nails by self		
10.	Comb and tie hairs by self		
11.	Able to move independently		
12.	Able to sit down in chair/bed by self		
13.	Able to climb stairs		
	Household Tasks		
14.	Perform routine household work (e.g. bed making, arranging furniture)		
15.	Wash clothes		

contd…

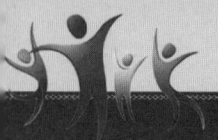
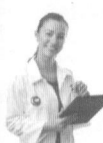

S. No.	Daily living activities	Yes/No
16.	Cooking	
17.	Keep living place clean and tidy	
18.	Open or close doors and windows of living room	
19.	Go to the market	
20.	Manage finances	
21.	Gardening	
	Outside Tasks	
22.	Meaningful leisure time activities (e.g. reading newspapers, social/religious gathering)	
23.	Go for an outing	
24.	Verbally communicate with relatives and friends	
25.	Communicate in writing (e.g. writing letters) with relatives/friends	
26.	Go to the temple/religious places	
27.	Go to a long distance for shopping	
28.	Go to the doctor/clinic	
29.	Go to the bank	
30.	Go do full time/part time job	

RISK OF ACCIDENT/INJURIES IN SURROUNDING ENVIRONMENT

S. No.	Risk of accident/injuries	Yes/No
1.	Slippery floor	
2.	Stagnant water on floor/bathroom	
3.	Inadequate lighting in passages/stairs/living room/bathroom	
4.	Furniture/objects in the passages or corridors	
5.	High height beds/Bed without side rails	
6.	High heeled/loose fitting shoes/slippers	
7.	No hearing aid with poor hearing acuity/Non-working hearing aid	
8.	No spectacles with blurred vision/Wearing new spectacles	
9.	Inability to recognize the temperature of water before bath/drink/hot water bottles	
10.	Keeping the medications or drinks unlabeled/near to the poisonous substances	

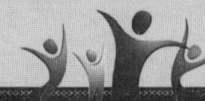

LAB INVESTIGATIONS

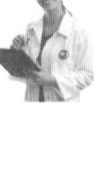

S. No.	Date/time	Investigation	Patient value	Normal value	Remarks

MEDICATIONS

S. No.	Name and action	Dose/route/frequency	Indication	Side effects

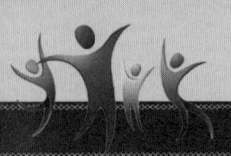 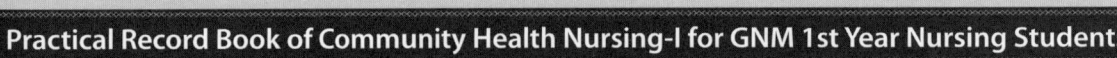
DIET CHART

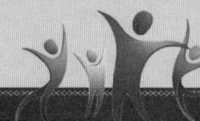

Identified Health Problems/Needs

_____
_____
_____
_____
_____
_____
_____
_____
_____

Prioritization of Health Problems/Needs

_____
_____
_____
_____
_____
_____
_____
_____
_____
_____

Priority Nursing Diagnosis

_____
_____
_____
_____
_____
_____
_____
_____
_____

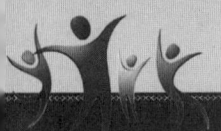

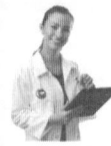

NURSING CARE PLAN

Assessment	Diagnosis	Goal/ Objective	Planning	Implementation	Evaluation

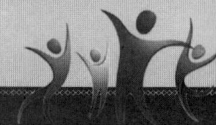

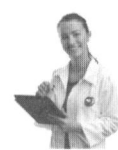

NURSING CARE PLAN

Assessment	Diagnosis	Goal/ Objective	Planning	Implementation	Evaluation

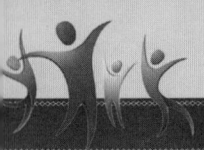

HEALTH EDUCATION

(Include diet/medication and its side effects/exercise/rest/self-care/hygiene/follow-up)

_____
_____
_____
_____
_____
_____
_____
_____
_____
_____
_____
_____
_____
_____
_____
_____
_____
_____

REFERENCES

_____
_____
_____
_____
_____
_____

Signature of Student   **Signature of Supervisor**

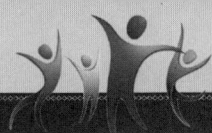

4. Health Education

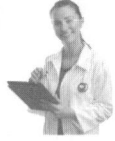

4.1. Urban

ON

_____

IDENTIFICATION DATA

Name of the Health Educator: _____

Health Education Topic _____

Age Group/Participants: _____

Size of the Group: _____

Date of Teaching: _____

Time of Teaching: _____

Duration of Teaching: _____

Place of Teaching: _____

Method of Teaching: _____

Teaching Aids: _____

Medium of Teaching/Language: _____

Name of the Student's Supervisor: _____

Self-Introduction

_____
_____
_____
_____
_____

Topic Introduction

_____
_____
_____
_____
_____
_____

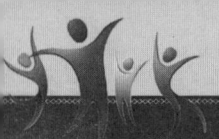

Previous Knowledge of the Group

_____

_____

_____

_____

_____

_____

_____

_____

_____

General Objective

_____

_____

_____

Specific Objectives

_____

_____

_____

_____

_____

_____

_____

_____

_____

_____

_____

_____

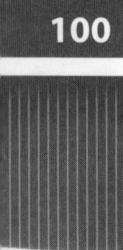

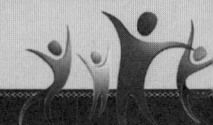

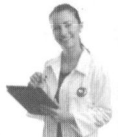

Time	Specific Objectives	Content	Health Educator Teaching Activity	A-V Aids	Participant's Evaluation

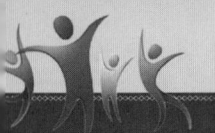

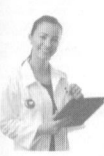

Time	Specific Objectives	Content	Health Educator Teaching Activity	A-V Aids	Participant's Evaluation

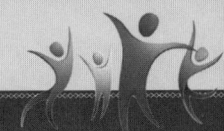
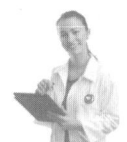

Time	Specific Objectives	Content	Health Educator Teaching Activity	A-V Aids	Participant's Evaluation

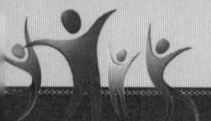
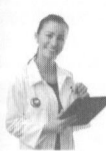

Time	Specific Objectives	Content	Health Educator Teaching Activity	A-V Aids	Participant's Evaluation

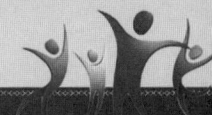
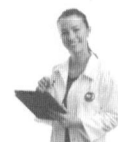

Time	Specific Objectives	Content	Health Educator Teaching Activity	A-V Aids	Participant's Evaluation

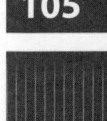

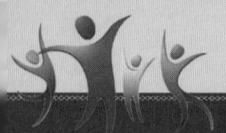

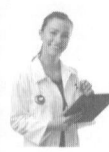

Time	Specific Objectives	Content	Health Educator Teaching Activity	A-V Aids	Participant's Evaluation

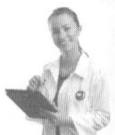

Time	Specific Objectives	Content	Health Educator Teaching Activity	A-V Aids	Participant's Evaluation

REFERENCES

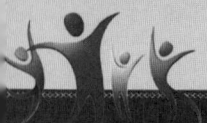
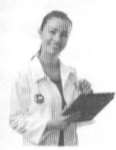

4.2. Rural

ON

_____

IDENTIFICATION DATA

Name of the Health Educator: _____

Health Education Topic _____

Age Group/Participants: _____

Size of the Group: _____

Date of Teaching: _____

Time of Teaching: _____

Duration of Teaching: _____

Place of Teaching: _____

Method of Teaching: _____

Teaching Aids: _____

Medium of Teaching/Language: _____

Name of the Student's Supervisor: _____

Self-Introduction

_____

_____

_____

_____

_____

Topic Introduction

_____

_____

_____

_____

_____

_____

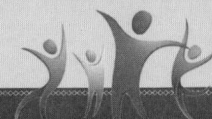

Previous Knowledge of the Group

_____

_____

_____

_____

_____

_____

_____

_____

_____

General Objective

_____

_____

_____

_____

Specific Objectives

_____

_____

_____

_____

_____

_____

_____

_____

_____

_____

_____

_____

_____

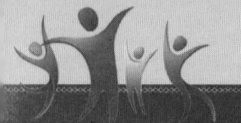

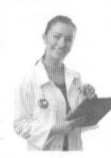

Time	Specific Objectives	Content	Health Educator Teaching Activity	A-V Aids	Participant's Evaluation

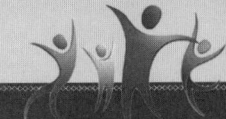

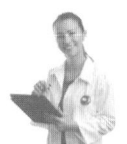

Time	Specific Objectives	Content	Health Educator Teaching Activity	A-V Aids	Participant's Evaluation

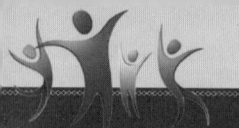

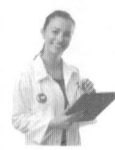

Time	Specific Objectives	Content	Health Educator Teaching Activity	A-V Aids	Participant's Evaluation

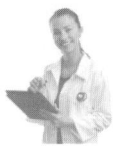

Time	Specific Objectives	Content	Health Educator Teaching Activity	A-V Aids	Participant's Evaluation

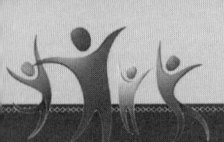

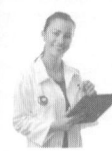

Time	Specific Objectives	Content	Health Educator Teaching Activity.	A-V Aids	Participant's Evaluation

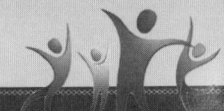

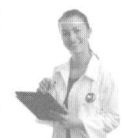

Time	Specific Objectives	Content	Health Educator Teaching Activity	A-V Aids	Participant's Evaluation

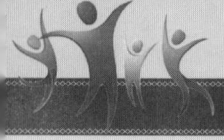

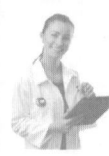

Time	Specific Objectives	Content	Health Educator Teaching Activity	A-V Aids	Participant's Evaluation

REFERENCES

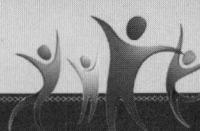

5. Nutritional Assessment

IDENTIFICATION DATA

Name: _____

Address: _____

Age/Sex: _____

Religion—Hindu/Muslims/Sikh/Christian/Others: _____

Caste—GEN/SC/ST/OBC: _____

Occupation—Unemployed/government/private job/Self-employed/daily wage worker/homemaker/others: _____

Region—North/South/East/West: _____

Level of activity—Sedentary/moderate/heavy worker: _____

Relation with head of the family: _____

Family size (Total Members): _____

Family income per capita (₹): _____

Nearby Sub-center/PHC/CHC/District Hospital: _____

FAMILY COMPOSITION AND CHARACTERISTICS

S. No.	Name of the family members	Relationship with head of the family	Date of Birth/ Sex (Male-M/ Female-F/ Transgender-T)	Marital Status (Unmarried/ Married)	Educa-tional status	Occup-ation	Monthly income (₹)	Dietary habits (Veg/ Non-veg)	Addiction (Smoking Alcohol/ Drugs/ Others)	Health status (Healthy/ unhealthy)
1.										
2.										
3.										
4.										
5.										
6.										
7.										
8.										

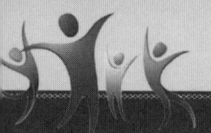

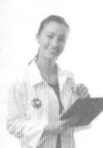

Food purchasing place: Market/local shop/weekly market places/others, specify_____

Household food production: No/vegetable garden/fruit tree/agriculture land/others, specify_____

Domestic animals: No/cow/buffalo/goat/pig/others, specify_____

Poultry: No/hen/duck/others, specify_____

Raw food preservation: No store/kitchen/store room/living room/others, specify_____

Cooked food preservation: No storage/kitchen/cup-board/refrigerator/others, specify_____

Type of cooking fuel: LPG/electric heater/kerosene stove/firewood/others, specify_____

Kitchen/cooking place: Clean/dirty_____

Number of meals per day_____

Anthropometric Measurement (In children)

Weight _____kg   Length/Height _____ cm   MAC_____cm   CC_____cm   HC_____cm

Degree of Malnutrition

$$\text{Weight for age} = \frac{\text{Actual weight of the child}}{\text{Expected weight of the child}} \times 100 = \underline{\hspace{6cm}}$$

Classification According to IAP

Weight for Age	Classification of under nutrition	In child
≥80%	Normal	Yes/No
71–80%	Grade-I	Yes/No
61–70%	Grade-II	Yes/No
51–60%	Grade-III	Yes/No
≤50%	Grade-IV	Yes/No

According to WHO Growth Charts

Weight for Age (0–3 Years)

Normal	Moderately Underweight (Below -2SD to 3SD)	Severely Underweight (Below 3SD)
Yes/No	Yes/No	Yes/No

Mid-Arm Circumference (7 Months–60 Months)

<11.5 cm (Red)	11.5–12.5 cm (Yellow)	≥12.5 cm (Green)
Yes/No	Yes/No	Yes/No

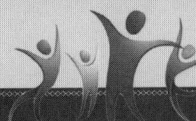
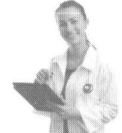

Anthropometric Measurement (In Adults)

Weight _____kg   Height _____ cm

BMI (Quetelet's Index) _____   [Weight (kg)/height^2 (meter)]

Interpretation of BMI: Underweight/normal/overweight/obese

Family Dietary Pattern

Food groups	Food items	Food consumption (yes/no)	Frequency of consumption (daily/ bi-weekly/ weekly/ monthly/ seasonally)	Average daily intake (in grams)	Expenditure per day (₹)	Method/Form of food preparation (boiling/steaming/ pressure cooking/ frying/baking/ germination/roasting/ fermentation)	Method of food storage at home (hygienic/ unhygienic)
Energy giving foods	Rice						
	Wheat						
	Tubers/roots						
	Edible oil						
	Ghee/butter						
	Dalda						
	Sugar/jaggery						
	Others						
Body building foods	Pulses						
	Meat						
	Fish						
	Poultry						
	Eggs						
	Others						
Protective foods	Vegetables						
	Fruits						
	Milk & milk products						
	Others						
Beverages	Tea						
	Coffee						
Others	Junk food						

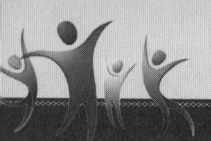

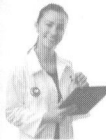

PHYSICAL ASSESSMENT FOR COMMON NUTRITIONAL DEFICIENCIES

Site	Abnormal Signs	Possible Nutritional Deficiency	Remarks
Appearance	Thin/sick Obese	Undernutrition Overnutrition	
Growth	Low weight/stunted growth	Protein/Energy/Zinc	
Skin	Dry and scaly/flaky/rough Delayed wound healing Dermatitis	Vitamin –A/Essential Fatty Acids Vitamin –C Niacin	
Hair	Thin and sparse/dry/lusterless/ Depigmentation/easily pluckable	Protein/Energy	
Face	Pale Edema/moon face	Iron/Vitamin-B6/B-12/Folate Protein	
Eyes	Pale Night blindness/Bitot's spot/ xerophthalmia	Iron Vitamin-A	
Lips	Cracked around corners Swelling/puffiness	Iron/Riboflavin/Niacin/Vitamin-B6 Riboflavin/Niacin	
Tongue	Pale	Iron/Vitamin B-12/Folic Acid	
Teeth	Mottled enamel/dental caries Discoloration	Excess Sugar Intake/Poor Dental Hygiene Dental Fluorosis	
Gums	Swelling/bleeding	Vitamin C (Ascorbic Acid)	
Neck	Thyroid gland enlargement	Iodine (Goiter)	
Nails	Pale/spoon shaped/Brittle	Iron	
Muscles	Wasting	Protein/Energy	
Skeletal	Knock knees/bowed legs/pigeon chest/enlarged joints	Vitamin D/Calcium	

LAB INVESTIGATIONS

S. No.	Date/time	Investigation	Patient value	Normal Value	Remarks
		Hb Estimation Stool Examination Blood Smear			

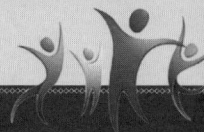
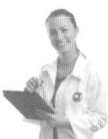

DIET CHART

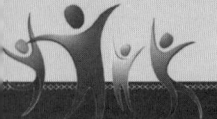
Identified Health Problems/Needs

_____
_____
_____
_____
_____
_____
_____
_____

Prioritization of Health Problems/Needs

_____
_____
_____
_____
_____
_____
_____
_____

Priority Nursing Diagnosis

_____
_____
_____
_____
_____
_____
_____
_____

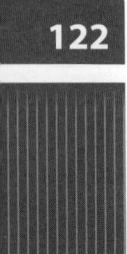

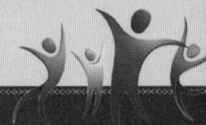

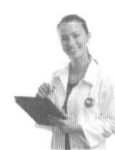

NURSING CARE PLAN

Assessment	Diagnosis	Goal/ Objective	Planning	Implementation	Evaluation

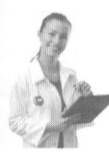

NURSING CARE PLAN

Assessment	Diagnosis	Goal/ Objective	Planning	Implementation	Evaluation

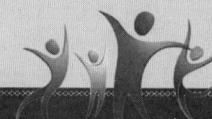
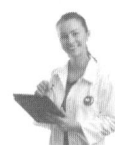

NURSING CARE PLAN

Assessment	Diagnosis	Goal/ Objective	Planning	Implementation	Evaluation

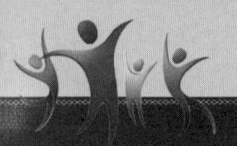

HEALTH EDUCATION

(Include diet-selection/purchasing/cooking/serving/preservation/consumption/food hygiene/follow-up)

_____

_____

_____

_____

_____

_____

_____

_____

_____

_____

_____

_____

_____

_____

_____

_____

_____

_____

_____

_____

REFERENCES

_____

_____

_____

_____

_____

_____

_____

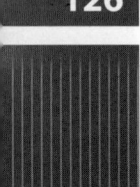

Signature of Student   **Signature of Supervisor**

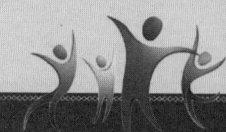

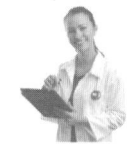

GROWTH CHART – BOY (0–3 YEARS)

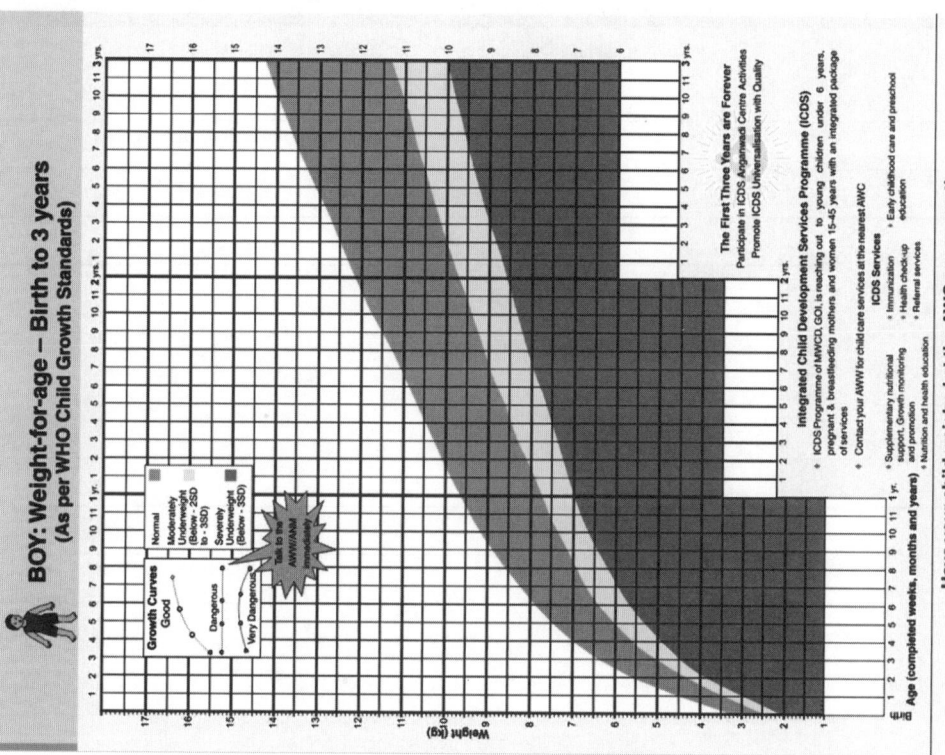

GROWTH CHART – GIRL (0–3 YEARS)

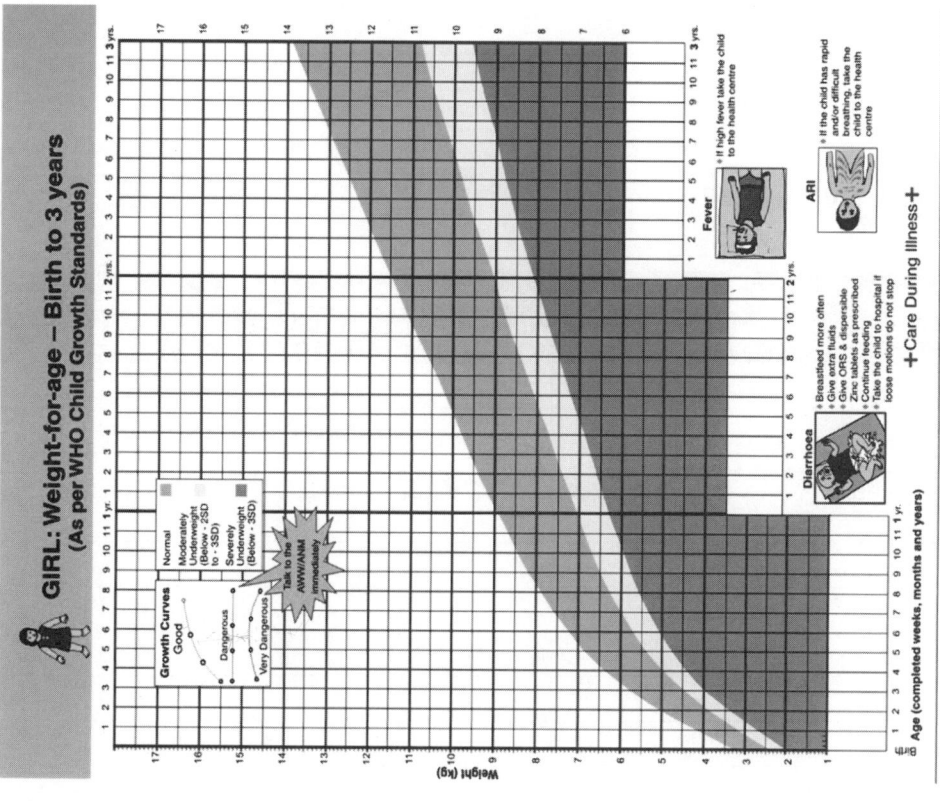

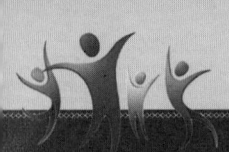

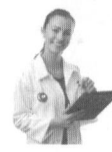

6. Nutritious Food Preparation/Cooking Demonstration

Name of the Recipe: _____

Name of the Client: _____

Age group/Age/Sex: _____

Diagnosis/Chief Complaints/Indication: _____

INTRODUCTION

_____
_____
_____
_____

OBJECTIVES

_____
_____
_____
_____

INGREDIENTS AND NUTRITIVE VALUE

Ingredient	Quantity	Calories (kcal)	Carbohyd-rate (g)	Protein (g)	Fat (g)	Iron (mg)	Calcium (mg)	Other important nutrients				
Total												

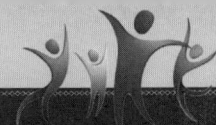

Price Calculation

S. No.	Ingredient	Price per kg Or per liter (₹)	Price as per amount used in Recipe (₹)
Total			₹

Steps of Preparation

_____

_____

_____

_____

_____

_____

_____

_____

_____

_____

Health Education

_____

_____

Feedback

_____

_____

References

_____

_____

Signature of Student

Signature of Supervisor

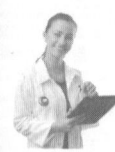

7. Procedure Demonstration

7.1. ....

IDENTIFICATION DATA

Name of the client: _____   Diagnosis: _____

Age/Sex: _____   Treatment (Taken/Not): _____

Chief complaints: _____   Indication/Need of procedure: _____

Definition

_____

_____

_____

Objectives/Need/Purpose

_____

_____

_____

_____

_____

_____

Preparation of the client

_____

_____

_____

Preparation of Articles

Article Name	Need/Purpose

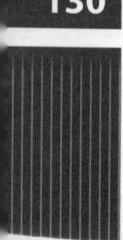

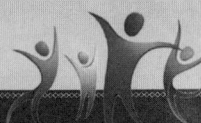

Steps of Procedure

After Care of the Client

After Care of the Articles

Documentation

Signature of Student

Signature of Supervisor

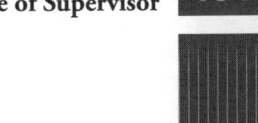

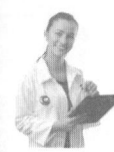

7.2. ....

IDENTIFICATION DATA

Name of the client: _____   Diagnosis: _____

Age/Sex: _____   Treatment (Taken/Not): _____

Chief complaints: _____   Indication/Need of procedure: _____

Definition

_____
_____
_____

Objectives/Need/Purpose

_____
_____
_____
_____
_____
_____

Preparation of the client

_____
_____
_____

Preparation of Articles

Article Name	Need/Purpose

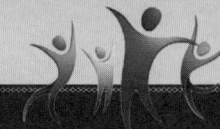

Steps of Procedure

_____

_____

_____

_____

_____

_____

_____

_____

_____

_____

_____

_____

_____

_____

_____

_____

_____

_____

After Care of the Client

_____

_____

_____

After Care of the Articles

_____

_____

_____

Documentation

_____

_____

_____

_____

Signature of Student   **Signature of Supervisor**

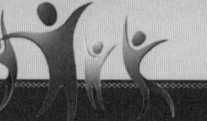

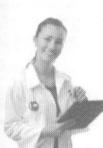

7.3. ....

IDENTIFICATION DATA

Name of the client: _____   Diagnosis: _____

Age/Sex: _____   Treatment (Taken/Not): _____

Chief complaints: _____   Indication/Need of procedure: _____

Definition

_____
_____
_____

Objectives/Need/Purpose

_____
_____
_____
_____
_____
_____

Preparation of the client

_____
_____
_____

Preparation of Articles

Article Name	Need/Purpose

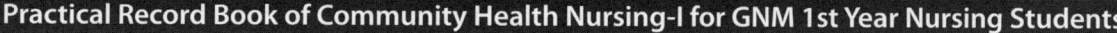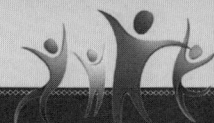
Steps of Procedure

_____
_____
_____
_____
_____
_____
_____
_____
_____
_____
_____
_____
_____
_____
_____
_____
_____
_____
_____

After Care of the Client

_____
_____
_____

After Care of the Articles

_____
_____
_____
_____

Documentation

_____
_____
_____
_____

Signature of Student   **Signature of Supervisor**

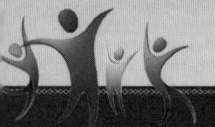

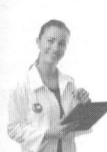

7.4. ....

IDENTIFICATION DATA

Name of the client: _____   Diagnosis: _____

Age/Sex: _____   Treatment (Taken/Not): _____

Chief complaints: _____   Indication/Need of procedure: _____

Definition

_____
_____
_____

Objectives/Need/Purpose

_____
_____
_____
_____
_____
_____

Preparation of the client

_____
_____
_____

Preparation of Articles

Article Name	Need/Purpose

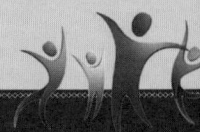

Steps of Procedure

_____
_____
_____
_____
_____
_____
_____
_____
_____
_____
_____
_____
_____
_____
_____
_____
_____
_____
_____
_____
_____
_____
_____

After Care of the Client

_____
_____
_____

After Care of the Articles

_____
_____
_____

Documentation

_____
_____
_____
_____

Signature of Student

Signature of Supervisor

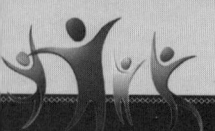
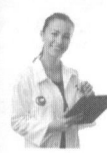

7.5. ....

IDENTIFICATION DATA

Name of the client: _____   Diagnosis: _____

Age/Sex: _____   Treatment (Taken/Not): _____

Chief complaints: _____   Indication/Need of procedure: _____

Definition

_____

_____

_____

Objectives/Need/Purpose

_____

_____

_____

_____

_____

_____

Preparation of the client

_____

_____

_____

Preparation of Articles

Article Name	Need/Purpose

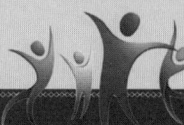

Steps of Procedure

_____

_____

_____

_____

_____

_____

_____

_____

_____

_____

_____

_____

_____

_____

_____

_____

_____

_____

_____

_____

_____

_____

After Care of the Client

_____

_____

_____

_____

After Care of the Articles

_____

_____

_____

_____

Documentation

_____

_____

_____

_____

Signature of Student   **Signature of Supervisor**

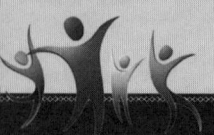
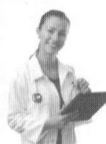

7.6. ....

IDENTIFICATION DATA

Name of the client: _____   Diagnosis: _____

Age/Sex: _____   Treatment (Taken/Not): _____

Chief complaints: _____   Indication/Need of procedure: _____

Definition

_____

_____

_____

Objectives/Need/Purpose

_____

_____

_____

_____

_____

_____

Preparation of the client

_____

_____

_____

Preparation of Articles

Article Name	Need/Purpose

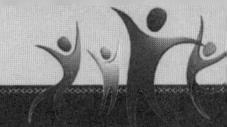

Steps of Procedure

_____

_____

_____

_____

_____

_____

_____

_____

_____

_____

_____

_____

_____

_____

_____

_____

_____

_____

_____

_____

_____

_____

After Care of the Client

_____

_____

_____

After Care of the Articles

_____

_____

_____

_____

Documentation

_____

_____

_____

_____

Signature of Student   **Signature of Supervisor**

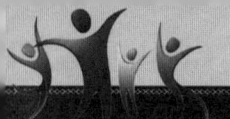

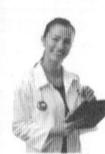

7.7. ....

IDENTIFICATION DATA

Name of the client: _____   Diagnosis: _____

Age/Sex: _____   Treatment (Taken/Not): _____

Chief complaints: _____   Indication/Need of procedure: _____

Definition

_____
_____
_____

Objectives/Need/Purpose

_____
_____
_____
_____
_____
_____

Preparation of the client

_____
_____
_____

Preparation of Articles

Article Name	Need/Purpose

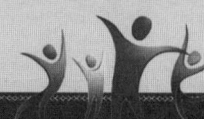

Steps of Procedure

_____
_____
_____
_____
_____
_____
_____
_____
_____
_____
_____
_____
_____
_____
_____
_____
_____

After Care of the Client

_____
_____
_____

After Care of the Articles

_____
_____
_____

Documentation

_____
_____
_____
_____

Signature of Student   **Signature of Supervisor**

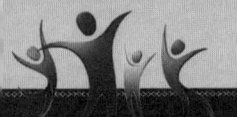

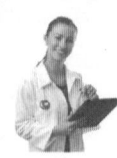

7.8. ....

IDENTIFICATION DATA

Name of the client: _____   Diagnosis: _____

Age/Sex: _____   Treatment (Taken/Not): _____

Chief complaints: _____   Indication/Need of procedure: _____

Definition

_____

_____

_____

Objectives/Need/Purpose

_____

_____

_____

_____

_____

Preparation of the client

_____

_____

_____

Preparation of Articles

Article Name	Need/Purpose

144

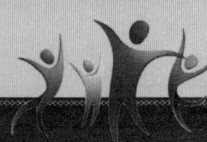

Steps of Procedure

_____
_____
_____
_____
_____
_____
_____
_____
_____
_____
_____
_____
_____
_____
_____
_____
_____
_____
_____

After Care of the Client

_____
_____
_____
_____

After Care of the Articles

_____
_____
_____
_____

Documentation

_____
_____
_____
_____

Signature of Student   **Signature of Supervisor**

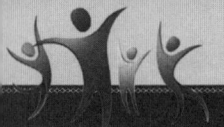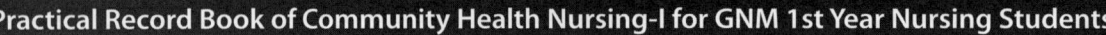

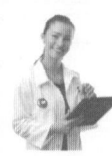

7.9. ....

IDENTIFICATION DATA

Name of the client: _____   Diagnosis: _____

Age/Sex: _____   Treatment (Taken/Not): _____

Chief complaints: _____   Indication/Need of procedure: _____

Definition

_____
_____
_____

Objectives/Need/Purpose

_____
_____
_____
_____
_____
_____

Preparation of the client

_____
_____
_____

Preparation of Articles

Article Name	Need/Purpose

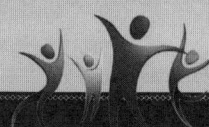

Steps of Procedure

_____

_____

_____

_____

_____

_____

_____

_____

_____

_____

_____

_____

_____

_____

_____

_____

_____

_____

After Care of the Client

_____

_____

_____

After Care of the Articles

_____

_____

_____

Documentation

_____

_____

_____

_____

Signature of Student

Signature of Supervisor

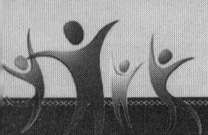
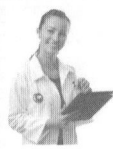

7.10. ....

IDENTIFICATION DATA

Name of the client: _____   Diagnosis: _____

Age/Sex: _____   Treatment (Taken/Not): _____

Chief complaints: _____   Indication/Need of procedure: _____

Definition

_____

_____

_____

Objectives/Need/Purpose

_____

_____

_____

_____

_____

_____

Preparation of the client

_____

_____

_____

Preparation of Articles

Article Name	Need/Purpose

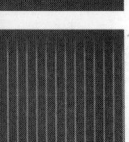

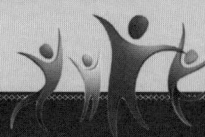

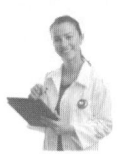

Steps of Procedure

_____

_____

_____

_____

_____

_____

_____

_____

_____

_____

_____

_____

_____

_____

_____

_____

_____

_____

_____

_____

_____

_____

_____

_____

After Care of the Client

_____

_____

_____

After Care of the Articles

_____

_____

_____

Documentation

_____

_____

_____

_____

Signature of Student   **Signature of Supervisor**

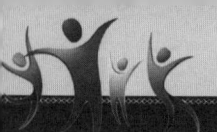

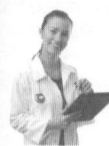

8. PREPARATION OF A-V AIDS

8.1. ....

_____

Introduction and Definition

_____
_____
_____
_____
_____
_____

Objectives of Preparation

_____
_____
_____
_____
_____
_____

Budget Calculation

S. No.	Article/material	Purpose	Quantity	Source of material (e.g. market/household waste etc.)	Money spent (₹)
Total					₹

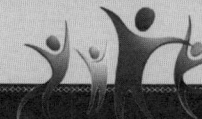
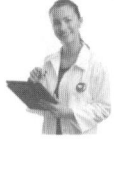

Steps of Preparation

_____
_____
_____
_____
_____
_____
_____
_____
_____

Paste a Picture/Draw a Diagram of Prepared A-V Aids

References

_____
_____

Signature of Student

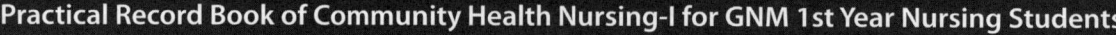

8.2. ....

_____

Introduction and Definition

_____
_____
_____
_____
_____
_____

Objectives of Preparation

_____
_____
_____
_____
_____
_____

Budget Calculation

S. No.	Article/material	Purpose	Quantity	Source of material (e.g. market/household waste etc.)	Money spent (₹)
Total					₹

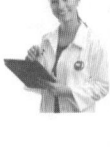

Steps of Preparation

_____

_____

_____

_____

_____

_____

_____

_____

Paste a Picture/Draw a Diagram of Prepared A-V Aids

References

_____

_____

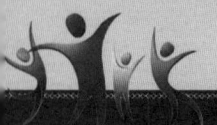

8.3. ....

Introduction and Definition

_____
_____
_____
_____
_____
_____

Objectives of Preparation

_____
_____
_____
_____
_____
_____

Budget Calculation

S. No.	Article/material	Purpose	Quantity	Source of material (e.g. market/household waste etc.)	Money spent (₹)
Total					₹

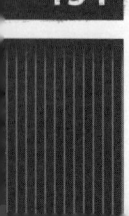

154

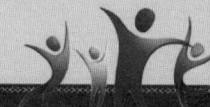
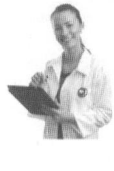

Steps of Preparation

_____

_____

_____

_____

_____

_____

_____

_____

Paste a Picture/Draw a Diagram of Prepared A-V Aids

References

_____

_____

Signature of Student

Signature of Supervisor

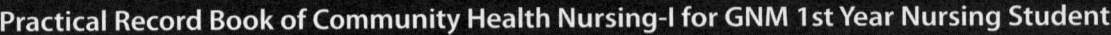
8.4. ....

_____

Introduction and Definition

_____
_____
_____
_____
_____
_____

Objectives of Preparation

_____
_____
_____
_____
_____
_____

Budget Calculation

S. No.	Article/material	Purpose	Quantity	Source of material (e.g. market/household waste etc.)	Money spent (₹)
Total					₹

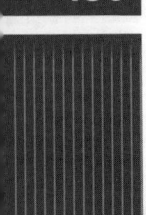

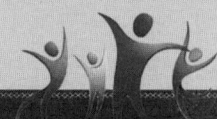

Steps of Preparation

_____

_____

_____

_____

_____

_____

_____

_____

Paste a Picture/Draw a Diagram of Prepared A-V Aids

References

_____

_____

Signature of Student

Signature of Supervisor

157

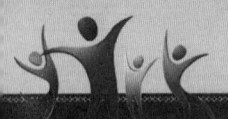

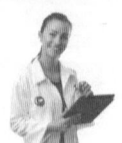

8.5. ....

_____

_____

Introduction and Definition

_____

_____

_____

_____

_____

_____

Objectives of Preparation

_____

_____

_____

_____

_____

_____

Budget Calculation

S. No.	Article/material	Purpose	Quantity	Source of material (e.g. market/household waste etc.)	Money spent (₹)
Total					₹

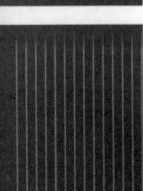

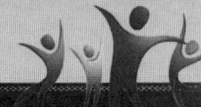

Steps of Preparation

_____

_____

_____

_____

_____

_____

_____

_____

Paste a Picture/Draw a Diagram of Prepared A-V Aids

References

_____

_____

Signature of Student

Signature of Supervisor

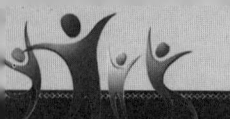
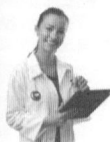

9. Set up of Different Clinics

9.1. ....

INTRODUCTION

_____

_____

_____

_____

_____

Date: _____

Venue: _____

Time: _____

Distance from College (in km): _____

Type of institution-Government/Private: _____

Name of the Student's Supervisor: _____

Objectives/Purpose: _____

_____

_____

_____

_____

Equipment and Resources

S. No.	Equipment/Resources	Quantity	Source/Supply/Funding

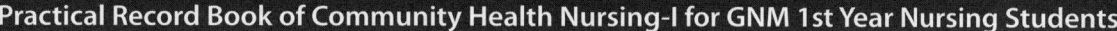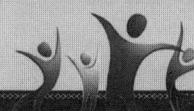

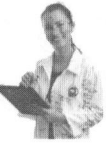

Health Personnel involvement in clinic/camp set-up

S. No.	Name of the Staff	Designation	Address of Hospital/Institute	Function

Steps/Method of organizing clinic/camp

_____
_____
_____
_____
_____
_____
_____
_____
_____
_____

Functions/Activities

_____
_____
_____
_____
_____
_____
_____
_____
_____
_____
_____
_____

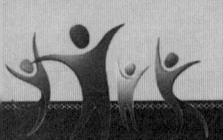
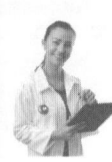

Map/floor plan showing the arrangement of stations/equipments/resources at clinic/camp

Records and reports maintained

_____
_____
_____
_____
_____
_____
_____
_____
_____

Student Nurse Learning

_____
_____
_____
_____

Signature of Student   Signature of Supervisor

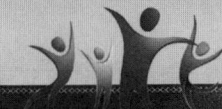

9.2. ....

INTRODUCTION

_____
_____
_____
_____
_____

Date: _____

Venue: _____

Time: _____

Distance from College (in km): _____

Type of institution-Government/Private: _____

Name of the Student's Supervisor: _____

Objectives/Purpose: _____
_____
_____
_____
_____

Equipment and Resources

S. No.	Equipment/Resources	Quantity	Source/Supply/Funding

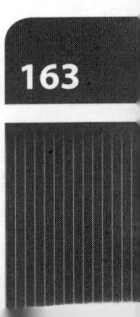

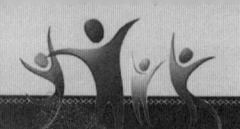

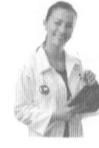

Health Personnel involvement in clinic/camp set-up

S. No.	Name of the Staff	Designation	Address of Hospital/Institute	Function

Steps/Method of organizing clinic/camp

_____

_____

_____

_____

_____

_____

_____

_____

_____

_____

Functions/Activities

_____

_____

_____

_____

_____

_____

_____

_____

_____

_____

_____

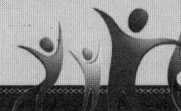

Map/floor plan showing the arrangement of stations/equipments/resources at clinic/camp

Records and reports maintained

_____
_____
_____
_____
_____
_____
_____
_____
_____
_____

Student Nurse Learning

_____
_____
_____
_____

Signature of Student

Signature of Supervisor

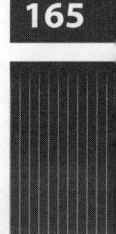

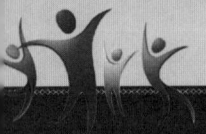

9.3. ....

INTRODUCTION

_____
_____
_____
_____
_____

Date: _____

Venue: _____

Time: _____

Distance from College (in km): _____

Type of institution-Government/Private: _____

Name of the Student's Supervisor: _____

Objectives/Purpose: _____

_____
_____
_____
_____

Equipment and Resources

S. No.	Equipment/Resources	Quantity	Source/Supply/Funding

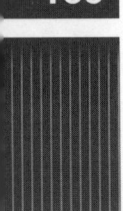

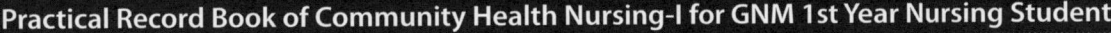
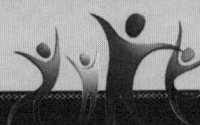

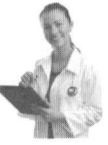

Health Personnel involvement in clinic/camp set-up

S. No.	Name of the Staff	Designation	Address of Hospital/Institute	Function

Steps/Method of organizing clinic/camp

_____

_____

_____

_____

_____

_____

_____

_____

_____

_____

Functions/Activities

_____

_____

_____

_____

_____

_____

_____

_____

_____

_____

_____

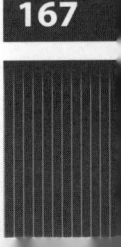

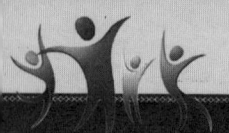
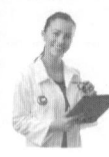

Map/floor plan showing the arrangement of stations/equipments/resources at clinic/camp

Records and reports maintained

_____
_____
_____
_____
_____
_____
_____
_____
_____

Student Nurse Learning

_____
_____
_____
_____

Signature of Student

Signature of Supervisor

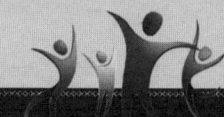

9.4. ....

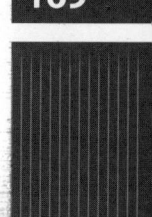

INTRODUCTION

_____
_____
_____
_____
_____
_____

Date: _____

Venue: _____

Time: _____

Distance from College (in km): _____

Type of institution-Government/Private: _____

Name of the Student's Supervisor: _____

Objectives/Purpose: _____
_____
_____
_____
_____

Equipment and Resources

S. No.	Equipment/Resources	Quantity	Source/Supply/Funding

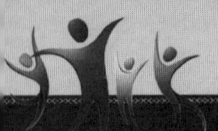

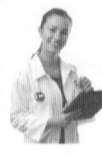

Health Personnel involvement in clinic/camp set-up

S. No.	Name of the Staff	Designation	Address of Hospital/Institute	Function

Steps/Method of organizing clinic/camp

_____

_____

_____

_____

_____

_____

_____

_____

Functions/Activities

_____

_____

_____

_____

_____

_____

_____

_____

_____

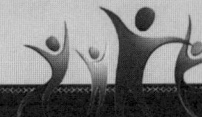

Map/floor plan showing the arrangement of stations/equipments/resources at clinic/camp

Records and reports maintained

_____
_____
_____
_____
_____
_____
_____
_____
_____
_____

Student Nurse Learning

_____
_____
_____
_____

Signature of Student

Signature of Supervisor

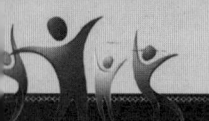

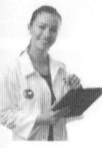

10. Observational Visits at Health and Welfare Agencies

10.1. Water Purification Plant

INTRODUCTION

_____

_____

_____

_____

Date: _____

Venue: _____

Time: _____

Distance from College (in km): _____

Name of the Head of the Water Purification Plant: _____

Type of Institution-Government/Private: _____

Name of the Student's Supervisor: _____

Visit Objectives

_____

_____

_____

_____

Organization Structure/Staffing Pattern

_____

_____

_____

_____

_____

_____

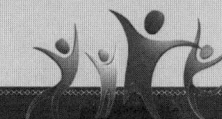

Area Map/Physical Set-up (Floor Plan) of the Water Purification Plant

Keys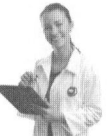

Components/Parts/Chambers

_____

_____

_____

_____

Procedure of Water Purification

_____

_____

_____

_____

_____

_____

_____

_____

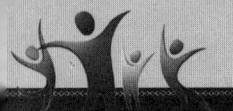

_____
_____
_____
_____
_____
_____
_____
_____
_____
_____
_____

Source of Funding

_____
_____
_____
_____

Records and Reports Maintained

_____
_____
_____
_____

Learning from the Visit for the Student Nurse

_____
_____
_____
_____

Signature of Student   **Signature of Supervisor**

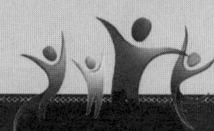
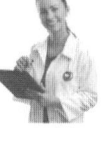

10.2. Sewage Purification Plant

INTRODUCTION

_____

_____

_____

_____

Date: _____

Venue: _____

Time: _____

Distance from College (in km): _____

Name of the Head of Sewage Purification Plant: _____

Type of Institution-Government/Private: _____

Name of the Student's Supervisor: _____

Visit Objectives

_____

_____

_____

_____

Organization Structure/Staffing Pattern

_____

_____

_____

_____

_____

_____

_____

_____

_____

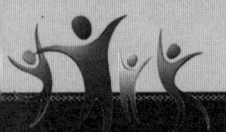

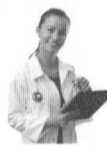

Area Map/Physical Set-up (Floor Plan) of the Sewage Purification Plant Keys

Components/Parts/Chambers

_____

_____

_____

_____

Procedure of Sewage Purification

_____

_____

_____

_____

_____

_____

_____

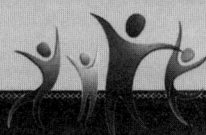

_____

_____

_____

_____

_____

_____

_____

_____

_____

_____

_____

Source of Funding

_____

_____

_____

_____

Records and Reports Maintained

_____

_____

_____

_____

Learning from the Visit for the Student Nurse

_____

_____

_____

_____

Signature of Student

Signature of Supervisor

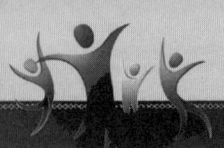
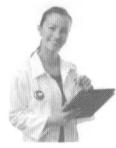

10.3. Milk Dairy
Observational/Orientation Visit

INTRODUCTION

_____
_____
_____
_____

Date: _____

Venue: _____

Time: _____

Distance from College (in km): _____

Name of the Head of the Milk Dairy: _____

Type of Institution-Government/Private: _____

Name of the Student's Supervisor: _____

Visit Objectives

_____
_____
_____
_____

Organization Structure/Staffing Pattern

_____
_____
_____
_____
_____
_____
_____

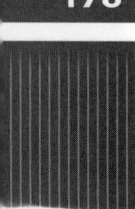

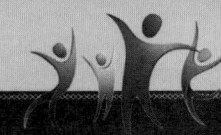

Area Map/Physical Set-up (Floor Plan) of the Milk Dairy

Keys

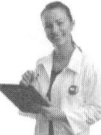

Components/Parts/Chambers

_____
_____
_____
_____

Procedure of Pasteurization of Milk

_____
_____
_____
_____
_____
_____
_____

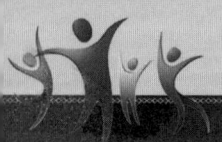

_____

_____

_____

_____

_____

_____

_____

_____

_____

_____

_____

Source of Funding

_____

_____

_____

_____

Records and Reports Maintained

_____

_____

_____

_____

Student Nurse Learning from the Visit

_____

_____

_____

_____

Signature of Student   **Signature of Supervisor**

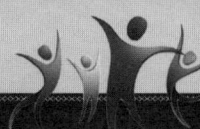
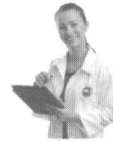

10.4. Panchayat
Observational/Orientation Visit

INTRODUCTION

_____
_____
_____
_____

Date: _____

Venue: _____

Time: _____

Distance from College (in km): _____

Name of the Sarpanch/Panchayat: _____

Name of the Student's Supervisor: _____

Visit Objectives

_____
_____
_____
_____

Organization Structure/Staffing Pattern

_____
_____
_____
_____

Selection Procedure of Panchayat Members

_____
_____
_____

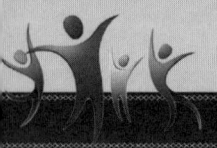
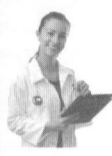

Area Map/Physical Set-up (Floor Plan) of the Panchayat Building   Keys

Department/Areas

_____

_____

_____

_____

Activities/Functions of Panchayat

_____

_____

_____

_____

_____

_____

_____

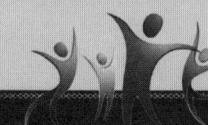

Social Welfare/Health Schemes Facilitated by Panchayat

1. Women (Antenatal/Postnatal/Widow)
   _____
   _____

2. Children
   _____
   _____

3. Adolescent Girls
   _____
   _____

4. Elderly
   _____
   _____

5. BPL Families
   _____
   _____

Source of Funding

_____
_____
_____
_____

Records and Reports Maintained

_____
_____
_____
_____

Learning from the Visit for the students Nurse

_____
_____
_____
_____

Signature of Student

Signature of Supervisor

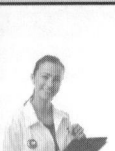

10.5. Any Other Community Organization

INTRODUCTION

_____

_____

_____

_____

Date: _____

Venue: _____

Time: _____

Distance from College (in km): _____

Name of the Head of the Institution: _____

Type of Institution-Government/Private: _____

Name of the Student's Supervisor: _____

Visit Objectives

_____

_____

_____

_____

Organization Structure/Staffing Pattern

_____

_____

_____

_____

_____

_____

_____

_____

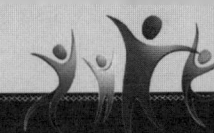

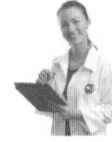

Physical Set-up (Floor Plan) of the Organization

Departments/Areas Available

_____

_____

_____

_____

Source of Funding for the Organization

_____

_____

_____

_____

Functions/Activities of the Organization

_____

_____

_____

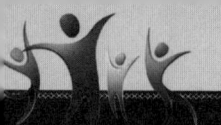

_____

_____

_____

_____

_____

_____

_____

_____

_____

Departments/Areas Available

_____

_____

_____

_____

Source of Funding for the Organization

_____

_____

_____

_____

Functions/Activities of the Organization

_____

_____

_____

_____

Signature of Student

Signature of Supervisor

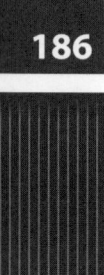

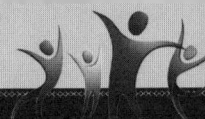

10.6. Any Other Community Organization

....

INTRODUCTION

_____

_____

_____

_____

Date: _____

Venue: _____

Time: _____

Distance from College (in km): _____

Name of the Head of the Institution: _____

Type of Institution-Government/Private: _____

Name of the Student's Supervisor: _____

Visit Objectives

_____

_____

_____

_____

Organization Structure/Staffing Pattern

_____

_____

_____

_____

_____

_____

_____

_____

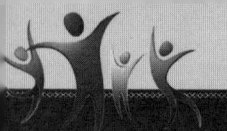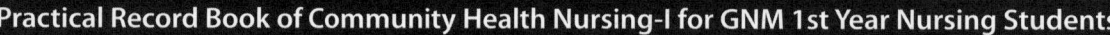

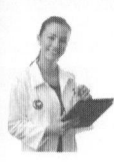 **Physical Set-up (Floor Plan) of the Organization**

Departments/Areas Available

_____

_____

_____

_____

Source of Funding for the Organization

_____

_____

_____

_____

Functions/Activities of the Organization

_____

_____

_____

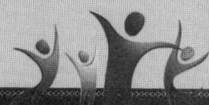

_____
_____
_____
_____
_____
_____
_____
_____
_____

Departments/Areas Available

_____
_____
_____
_____

Source of Funding for the Organization

_____
_____
_____
_____

Functions/Activities of the Organization

_____
_____
_____
_____

Signature of Student

Signature of Supervisor

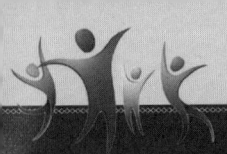

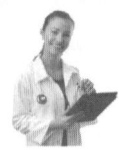

11. Home Visit and Family Folder

(Fill the family folders as per sample provided with the record book)

1. URBAN

Demographic Profile

Area: _____

Tehsil/Taluka: _____

Block: _____

District: _____

SC: _____

PHC: _____

CHC: _____

Family Folder Details

S.No	Date of issue	Name of head of the family	Address	Religion	Identified health needs	Interventions/ treatment	Date of submission	Signature of student	Signature of supervisor

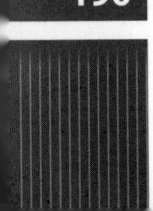

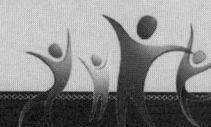
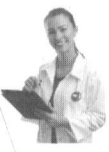

2. RURAL

Demographic Profile

Area: _____

Tehsil/Taluka: _____

Block: _____

District: _____

SC: _____

PHC: _____

CHC: _____

Family Folder Details

S. No.	Date of issue	Name of head of the family	Address	Religion	Identified health needs	Interventions/ treatment	Date of submission	Signature of student	Signature of supervisor

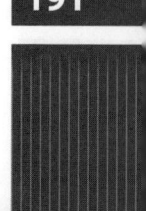

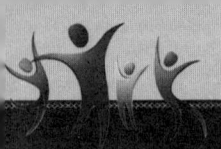

12. Assignments/Reports (Additional)

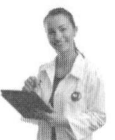

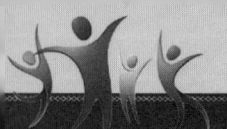

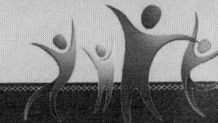

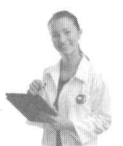

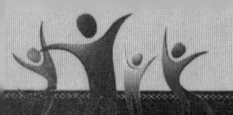

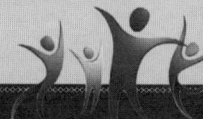
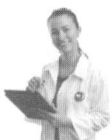

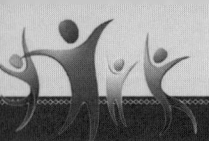

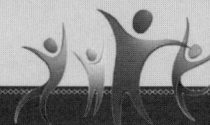

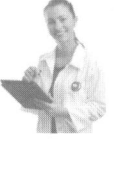

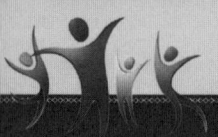

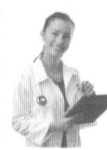

Annexures

NORMAL VALUES IN BLOOD INVESTIGATIONS

Blood investigations	Normal values
Hemoglobin	M: 13–17 g/dL F: 11–15 g/dL
White Blood Cell count	4.0–10x10³/μL
WBC Differential Segmented neutrophils Band neutrophils Lymphocytes Monocytes Eosinophils Basophils	 50–70% 0–8% 20–40% 4–8% 0–4% 0–2%
Reticulocytes count	0.5–1.5% of RBC
Erythrocytes sedimentation rate (ESR)	<30 mm/hr
Hematocrit	M: 39–50% F: 35–47%
Platelets (thrombocytes)	150– 400 × 10³/μL
Bleeding time	2–7 min
Activated partial thromboplastin time (aPTT)	25–35 sec
Prothrombin time (PT)	11–16 sec
Red blood indices Mean corpuscular volume (MCV) Mean corpuscular hemoglobin (MCH) Mean corpuscular hemoglobin concentration (MCHC)	 80–100 fL 27–34 pg 32–37%
Blood urea	13–43 mg/dL
Serum creatinine	0.6–1.3 mg/dL
Serum Albumin	3.5–5.0 g/dL
Sodium	135–145 mEq/L
Potassium	3.5–5.0 mEq/L
Calcium	8.6–10.2 mg/dL
Cholesterol High-density lipoproteins (HDLs) Low-density lipoproteins (LDLs)	<200 mg/dL M:- >40 mg/dL Fe:- >50 mg/dL Recommended: <100 mg/dL
Bilirubin Total Indirect Direct	 0.2–1.2 mg/dL 0.1–1.0 mg/dL 0.1–0.3 mg/dL
Acetone Quantitative Qualitative	 <2.0 mg/dL Negative

contd...

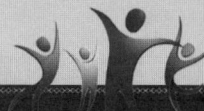
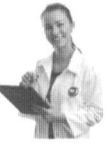

Blood investigations	Normal values
Ammonia	15–45 µgN/dl
Amylase	30–122 U/L
Lipase	31–186 U/L
Zinc	70–120 mcg/dL

NORMAL VALUES OF URINE INVESTIGATIONS

Urine investigations	Normal values
Acetone	Negative
Amylase	1–17 U/hr
Bilirubin	Negative
Calcium	100–250 mg/day
Creatine	<100 mg/day
Creatinine	0.6–2.0 g/day
Glucose	Negative
Hemoglobin	Negative
Ketone bodies	20–50 mg/day
Osmolality	300–1300 mOsm/kg
pH	4.0–8.0
Protein	0-trace
Sodium	40–220 mEq/day
Specific gravity	1.003–1.030
Uric acid	250–750 mg/day

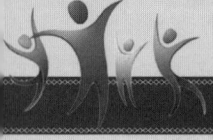 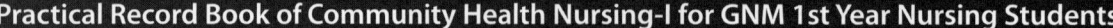

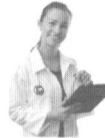

WHO RECOMMENDED NUTRITIVE VALUES FOR COMMONLY USED FOOD ITEM IN INDIA

Food Stuffs	Amount	Proteins (g)	Fats (g)	CHO (g)	Energy (kcal)
Milk and Milk Products					
Milk toned	100 cc	3.5	3.5	5.0	66
Milk cow's	100 cc	3.2	4.1	4.4	67
Milk goat's	100 cc	3.3	4.5	4.6	72
Milk buffalo's	100 cc	4.3	6.5	5.0	117
Milk human	100 cc	1.1	3.4	7.4	65
Curds	100 cc	3.1	4.0	3.0	60
Curds toned	100 cc	3.0	3.0	4.0	55
Butter milk	100 cc	0.8	1.1	0.5	15
Milk powder	100 g	38.0	0.1	51.0	357
Milk liquid	100 cc	2.5	0.1	4.6	29
Paneer	100 g	18.3	20.8	1.2	265
Cheese processed	100 g	24.0	25.1	6.3	348
Whole milk powder	100 g	25.8	26.7	38.0	496
Cream	100 g	1.5	40.0	2.5	385
Cereals and Pulses					
Wheat atta	100 g	12.1	1.7	69.4	341
Rice	100 g	6.8	0.5	78.2	345
Maize	100 g	11.1	3.6	66.2	342
Gram	100 g	17.0	5.3	61.0	360
Porridge	100 g	12.0	1.5	71.2	346
Oat meal	100 g	13.6	7.6	62.8	37.4
Cornflakes	100 g	0.8	-	85.0	385
Popcorns (salt added)	100 g	13.0	5.0	87.0	385
Rice flakes	100 g	6.6	1.2	77.3	346
Rice puffed (salt added)	100 g	7.5	0.1	73.6	325
Suji	100 g	10.4	0.8	74.8	348
Vermicelli/Semiya	100 g	8.7	0.4	78.3	352
Maida	100 g	11.0	0.9	73.9	348
Corn flour or custard powder	100 g	0.5	-	86.6	345
Biscuit sweet	100 g	6.4	15.2	71.9	450
Bengal gram whole	100 g	17.1	5.3	60.9	360
Dal chana	100 g	20.8	5.6	59.8	372
Black gram dal	100 g	24.0	1.4	59.6	347
Urad dal washed	100 g	24.0	1.5	60.0	350
Green gram dal	100 g	24.5	1.2	59.9	348
Green gram whole	100 g	24.0	1.3	56.7	334
Lentil (masoor dal)	100 g	25.0	0.7	59.0	343
Red gram dal (Arhar)	100 g	22.3	1.7	57.6	335

 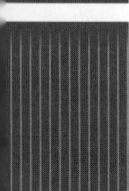

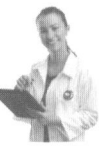

Food Stuffs	Amount	Proteins (g)	Fats (g)	CHO (g)	Energy (kcal)
Peas dried	100 g	19.7	1.1	56.5	315`
Rajma	100 g	23.0	1.3	60.6	346
Soya bean	100 g	43.2	19.5	20.9	432
Meat and Poultry					
Egg	100 g	13.3	13.3	-	173
Egg	1	6.6	6.6	-	76
Egg yolk	100 g	3.3	6.0	-	67
Egg white	100 g	3.0	-	-	12
Mutton (muscle)	100 g	18.5	13.3	-	194
Mutton (bone)	100 g	14.5	11.0	-	158
Fish	100 g	17.0	1.3	1.8	87
Chicken with bone	100 g	16.0	5.0	-	70
Chicken with muscle	100 g	25.0	0.5	-	109
Liver (goat)	100 g	20.0	3.0	-	107
Pork	100 g	18.7	4.4	-	114
Pigeon	100 g	23.3	4.9	-	137
Vegetables					
Cabbage	100 g	1.8	0.1	4.6	27
Coriander leaves	100 g	3.3	0.6	6.3	44
Curry leaves	100 g	6.1	1.0	18.7	108
Drum sticks	100 g	2.5	0.1	3.7	26
Fenugreek (methi)	100 g	4.4	0.9	6.0	49
Radish leaves	100 g	3.8	0.4	2.4	28
Lettuce	100 g	2.1	0.3	2.5	21
Mint	100 g	4.8	0.6	5.8	48
Mustard leaves (sarson)	100 g	4.0	0.6	3.2	34
Spinach	100 g	2.0	0.7	2.9	26
Carrot	100 g	0.9	0.2	10.6	48
Colocasia	100 g	3.0	0.1	21.1	97
Beet root	100 g	1.7	0.1	8.8	43
Onion	100 g	1.2	-	11.0	50
Onion small	100 g	1.8	0.1	12.6	59
Potato	100 g	1.6	0.1	22.6	97
Radish	100 g	0.7	0.1	3.4	17
Sweet potato	100 g	1.2	0.3	28.2	120
Turnip	100 g	0.5	0.2	6.2	29
Yam	100 g	1.4	0.1	26.0	111
Bitter gourd (karela)	100 g	1.6	0.2	4.2	25
Ghia	100 g	0.2	0.1	2.5	12
Brinjal	100 g	1.4	0.3	4.0	24
Cauliflower	100 g	2.6	0.4	4.0	30

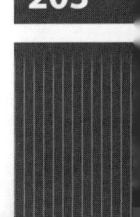

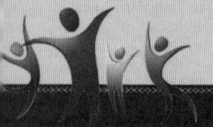

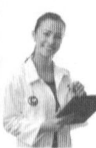

Food Stuffs	Amount	Proteins (g)	Fats (g)	CHO (g)	Energy (kcal)
French beans	100 g	1.7	0.1	4.5	26
Giant chillies	100 g	1.3	0.3	4.3	24
Kholkhol	100 g	1.1	0.2	3.8	21
Lady finger	100 g	1.9	0.2	6.4	35
Peas	100 g	7.2	0.1	15.9	93
Pumpkin	100 g	1.4	0.1	4.6	25
Tinda	100 g	1.4	0.2	3.4	21
Tomato green	100 g	1.9	0.1	3.6	23
Tomato ripe	100 g	0.9	0.2	3.6	20
Cucumber	100 g	0.4	0.1	2.5	13
Fruits					
Apple	100 g	0.2	0.5	13.4	59
Amla	100 g	0.1	0.5	13.7	58
Apricot dried	100 g	1.6	0.7	73.4	306
Bael fruit	100 g	1.8	0.3	31.8	137
Banana	100 g	1.2	0.3	27.2	116
Apricot fresh	100 g	1.0	0.3	11.6	53
Cherries red	100 g	1.1	0.5	13.8	64
Currants black	100 g	2.7	0.5	75.2	316
Dates dried	100 g	2.5	0.4	75.8	317
Guava	100 g	0.9	0.3	11.2	51
Grapes	100 g	0.5	0.3	16.5	71
Lemon	100 g	1.0	0.9	11.1	57
Jamun	100 g	0.7	0.3	14.0	62
Litchie	100 g	1.1	0.2	13.6	61
Lime sweet (Musambi)	100 g	0.8	0.3	9.3	43
Mango	100 g	0.6	0.4	16.9	74
Orange	100 g	0.7	0.2	10.9	48
Orange juice	100 g	0.2	0.1	1.9	9
Papaya ripe	100 g	0.6	0.1	7.2	32
Peaches	100 g	1.2	0.3	10.5	50
Pear	100 g	0.6	0.2	11.9	52
Plums	100 g	0.7	0.5	11.1	52
Pineapples	100 g	0.4	0.1	10.8	46
Pomegranate	100 g	1.6	0.1	14.5	65
Raspberry	100 g	1.0	0.6	11.6	56
Nuts and Oil Seeds					
Almond	100 g	20.8	58.9	10.5	655
Cashew nuts	100 g	21.2	46.9	22.3	596
Charoli seeds	100 g	19.0	59.0	12.0	666
Coconut dry	100 g	6.8	62.3	18.4	662

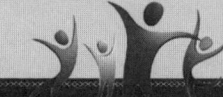

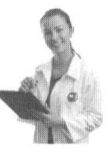

Food Stuffs	Amount	Proteins (g)	Fats (g)	CHO (g)	Energy (kcal)
Coconut fresh	100 g	4.5	41.6	13.0	444
Walnut	100 g	15.6	64.5	11.0	687
Gingelly seeds	100 g	18.3	43.3	25.0	563
Ground nuts	100 g	26.2	39.8	26.7	570
Pistachio nut	100 g	19.8	53.5	16.2	626
Chilgoza	100 g	13.9	49.3	29.0	615
Butter and Oils					
Butter	100 g	-	81.0	-	729
Ghee (pure)	100 g	-	100	-	900
Vege cooking oil	100 g	-	100	-	900
Vanaspati ghee	100 g	-	100	-	900
Miscellaneous food stuff					
Arrowroot	100 g	0.2	0.1	83.1	334
Betel leaves	100 g	3.1	0.8	6.1	44
Cane sugar	100 g	0.1	0	99.4	398
Honey	100 g	0.3	0	79.5	319
Jaggery	100 g	0.4	0.1	95.0	383
Papped	100 g	18.8	0.3	52.4	288
Sago	100 g	0.2	0.2	87.1	351
Yeast dried	100 g	39.5	0.6	391	320
Jam	30 g	0.1	-	18.0	73
Beer 6%	250 cc	-	-	4.0	110
Whiskey 42%	50 cc	-	-	-	140
Brandy 54%	50 cc	-	-	-	150
Horlicks	One tb. spoon	2.4	0.1	7	42
Horlicks	100 g	14.0	0.8	72	416
Bread	100 g	7.8	0.7	52	245

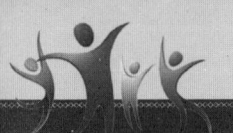
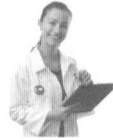

RECOMMENDED DIETARY ALLOWANCES (RDA) FOR VARIOUS CATEGORIES

Group	Particulars	Body wt (kg)	Net energy Kcal/d	Protein g/d	Visible fat g/day	Calcium mg/day	Iron mg/d	Vitamin-A retinol	Vitamin-A β-carotene	Thiamine mg/day	Riboflavin mg/d	Niacin equivalent	Pyridoxine mg/d	Ascorbic acid mg/d	Dietary folate µg/d	Vit-B$_{12}$ µg/d	Magnesium mg/d	Zinc mg/day
Man	Sedentary work	60	2320		25					1.2	1.4	16						
	Moderate work		2730	60.0	30	600	17	600	4800	1.4	1.6	18	2.0	40	200	1.0	340	12
	Heavy work		3490		40					1.7	2.1	21						
Woman	Sedentary work	55	1900		20					1.0	1.1	12						
	Moderate work		2230	55.0	25	600	21	600	4800	1.1	1.3	14	2.0	40	200	1.0	310	10
	Heavy work		2850		30					1.4	1.7	16						
	Pregnant		+350	82.2	30	1200	35	800	6400	+0.2	+0.3	+2	2.5	60	500	1.2		
	Lactation 0–6 m		+600	77.9	30	1200	25	950	7600	+0.3	+0.4	+4	2.5	80	500	1.5		12
	6–12 m		+520	70.2	30					+0.2	+0.3	+3	2.5					
Infants	0–6 m	5.4	92 kcal/kg/d	1.16 g/kg/d	—	500	46 µg/kg/d	350	—	0.2	0.3	710 µg/kg	0.1	25	25	0.2	30	—
	6–12 m	8.4	80 kcal/kg/d	1.69 g/kg/d	19	500	05		2800	0.3	0.4	650 µg/kg	0.4	25	25	0.2	45	—
Children	1–3 years	12.9	1060	16.7	27	600	09	400	3200	0.5	0.6	8	0.9	40	80	0.2–1.0	50	5
	4–6 years	18.0	1350	20.1	25		13	600	4800	0.7	0.8	11	0.9	40	100	0.2–1.0	70	7
	7–9 years	25.1	1690	29.5	30	600	16	600	4800	0.8	1.0	13	1.6	40	120	0.2–1.0	100	8
Boys	10–12 years	34.3	2190	39.9	35	800	21	600	4800	1.1	1.3	15	1.6	40	140	0.2–1.0	120	9
Girls	10–12 years	35.0	2010	40.4	35	800	27			1.0	1.2	13	1.6	40	140	0.2–1.0	160	9
Boys	13–15 years	47.6	2750	54.3	45	800	32			1.4	1.6	16	2.0	40	150		165	11
Girls	13–15 years	46.6	2330	51.9	40	800	27	600	4800	1.2	1.4	14	2.0	40	150	0.2–1.0	210	11
Boys	16–17 years	55.4	3020	61.5	50	800	28			1.5	1.8	17	2.0	40	200		195	12
Girls	16–17 years	52.1	2440	55.5	35	800	26			1.0	1.2	14	2.0	40	200	0.2–1.0	235	12

Source: *Indian Council of Medical Research 2010*

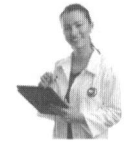

SUMMARY OF RECOMMENDED DIETARY ALLOWANCES (RDA) FOR ENERGY, PROTEIN, FAT AND MINERALS FOR INDIANS–2010

Group	Category/Age	Body weight (kg)	Net energy (kcal/kg/d)	Protein (g/kg/d)	Visible fat (g/d)	Calcium (mg/d)	Iron (mg/kg/d)	Zinc (mg/d)	Magnesium (mg/d)
Man	Sedentary work	60	2,320	60	25	600	17	12	340
	Moderate work		2,730		30				
	Heavy work		3,490		40				
Woman	Sedentary work	55	1,900	55	20	600	21	10	310
	Moderate work		2,230		25				
	Heavy work		2,850		30				
	Pregnant woman		+350	78	30	1,200	35	12	
	Lactation 0–6 months		+600	74	30	1,200	21		
	Lactation 6–12 months		+520	68	30				
Infants	0–6 months	5.4	92	1.16	–	500	46	–	30
	6–12 months	8.4	80	1.69	19		05	–	45
Children	1–3 years	12.9	1,060	16.7	27	600	09	5	50
	4–6 years	18.0	1,350	20.1	25		13	7	70
	7–9 years	25.1	1,690	29.5	30		16	8	100
Boys	10–12 years	34.3	2,190	39.9	35	800	21	9	120
Girls	10–12 years	35.0	2,010	40.4	35	800	27	9	160
Boys	13–15 years	47.6	2,750	54.3	45	800	32	11	165
Girls	13–15 years	46.6	2,330	51.9	40	800	27	11	210
Boys	16–17 years	55.4	3,020	61.5	50	800	28	12	195
Girls	16–17 years	52.1	2,440	55.5	35	800	26	12	235

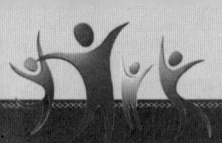

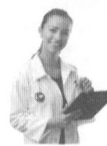

SOCIOECONOMIC SCALE

Socioeconomic Status Scales (India)

Rural	Udai Pareek , Modified BG Prasad, Shirpurkar, Radhuka
Urban	Modified Kuppuswamy Scale, Shrivastava, Jalota, Kulshreshtha, Gaurs

Table 1: Modified Kuppuswamy socioeconomic status Scale (India)

Education of head of family	Score
1. Professional degree or honors	7
2. Graduate or Postgraduate	6
3. Intermediate or Post High School Diploma	5
4. High School Certificate	4
5. Middle School Certificate	3
6. Primary School Certificate	2
7. Illiterate	1
Occupation of head of family	**Score**
1. Professional	10
2. Semi-professional	6
3. Clerical, shop-owner, farmer	5
4. Skilled worker	4
5. Semi-skilled worker	3
6. Unskilled worker	2
7. Unemployed	1
Total monthly family income (in ₹- Using Consumer Price Index on Jan 2017)	**Score**
≥42259	12
21130–42258	10
15847–21129	6
10565–15846	4
6339–10564	3
2134–6338	2
≤2133	1
Total Score	**Socioeconomic class**
26–29	Upper (I)
16–25	Upper middle (II)
11–15 middle	Lower-middle (III)
5–10 lower	Upper-lower (IV)
< 5	Lower (V)

Minimum Score = 3, Maximum Score = 29

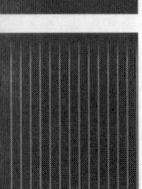

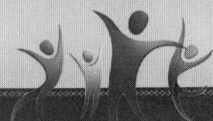
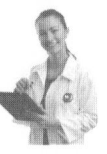

Table 2: Modified Pareek Rural Socioeconomic Status Scale

- Caste

  SC (1), Lower caste (2), Artisan caste (3), Agriculture caste (4), Prestige caste (5), Dominant caste (6).
- Occupation of head of family

  None (0), Laborer (1) Caste occupation (2), Business (3), Independent profession (4), Cultivation (5), Service (6)
- Education of head of family

  Illiterate (0), Can read only (1), Can read/write (2), Primary (3) Middle (4), High School (5), Graduate and above (6)
- Land holding

  No land (0), less than 1 acre (1), 1–5 acre (2), 5-10 acre (3), 10-15 acre (4), 15-20 acre (5), >20 acre (6).
- Social participation of head of family

  None (0), Member of one organization (like Panchayat, Nambardar etc.) (1), Member of >1 organization (2), Office holder in such organization (3), Wider public leader (6)
- Family Members Up to 5 (1), Above 5 (2)
- Level of Housing
- No House (1), Kutcha House (2), Mixed House (3), Pucca House (4) Mansion (6)
- Farm Power

  No. drought (buffalo/cow) animal (1), 1-2 drought animal (2), 3-4 drought animals (3), 5-6 drought animals or tractor (6)
- Material Possession

  Bullock cart (1), Cycle (1), Radio (1), Chairs (1), Improved agriculture equipments (2), none (0)

Figures in () brackets indicate scores

Socioeconomic class [pareek scale]	
Score more than 43	Class-I
Score 33–42	Class-II
Score 24–32	Class-III
Score 13–23	Class-IV
Score less than 13	Class-V

Table 3: BG Prasad Socioeconomic Scale

Socioeconomic class	Original classification (1960) –based on per capita family income in rupees	Updated based on per capita family in- come in rupees (2017)-method P Kumar
Class-I	100 and Above	6254 and Above
Class-II	50–99	3127–6253
Class-III	30–49	1876–3126
Class-IV	15–29	938–1875
Class-V	<15	<937

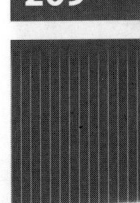

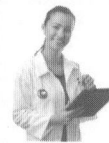
COMMUNITY NEED IDENTIFICATION AND VITAL STATISTICS SURVEY (PART-1)

General Information

Village/Area Name: _____

Panchayat: _____ Block: _____ Tehsil/Taluka: _____

District: _____

Total Population: _____

Total Families: _____

Fill the name of the organization and its distance from the community area in the space provided below

Nearby Health Care Facilities

District Hospital: _____

Government Maternity Hospital (if any): _____

Mission Hospital (if any): _____

Total Private Hospitals: _____

Subcenter: _____

Primary Health Center: _____

Community Health Center: _____

Indigenous medicine (hospital/clinic/dispensary)

- Ayurveda: _____
- Yoga: _____
- Naturopathy: _____
- Unani: _____
- Siddha: _____
- Homeopathy: _____
- If other, Specify: _____

Non-Governmental Organizations/Voluntary Health Organizations

- Orphan Age Children: _____
- Physically Challenged: _____
- Visually Challenged: _____
- Mentally Challenged: _____
- Hearing Challenged: _____
- Women: _____
- Elderly: _____
- Youth Welfare: _____
- Other: _____

Social Agencies

- Post Office: _____
- Bank: _____
- Police station: _____

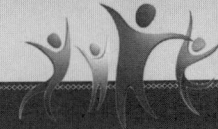
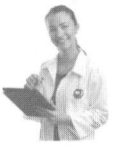

Religious Place

- Temple: _____
- Mosque: _____
- Gurudwara: _____
- Church: _____
- If others, Specify: _____

Education Facilities

Government

- Anganwadis: _____
- Balwadis: _____
- Primary School: _____
- Elementary School: _____
- Secondary School: _____
- Senior Secondary School: _____
- UG Institutions: _____
- PG Institutions: _____

Private

- Primary School: _____
- Elementary School: _____
- Secondary School: _____
- Senior Secondary School: _____
- UG Institutions: _____
- PG institutions: _____

Recreation Facilities

- Common Market Place: _____
- Playgrounds: _____
- Public Gardens: _____
- Cinema Halls: _____
- Clubs: _____
- Public Library: _____
- Fairs: _____
- Festivals: _____

Communication Facilities

- Post Office: _____
- Public Telephone Booths: _____
- Computer Center With Internet Facility: _____
- Traditional Media (Puppets, Folk Dance etc.): _____

Transport Facilities

- Railway Station:_____
- Bus Stand: _____
- Auto Stand: _____
- Taxi Stand: _____
- Airport: _____

Facilities for the Disposal of Dead Bodies: _____

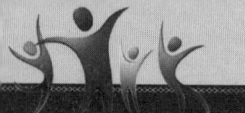

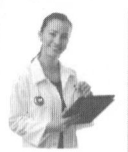

COMMUNITY NEED IDENTIFICATION AND VITAL STATISTICS SURVEY (PART-2)

Village/Area Name: _____ Tehsil/Taluka: _____ District: _____

2.1 SOCIO- DEMOGRAPHIC CHARACTERISTICS

General information			Age group								Sex			Religion				Caste				Marital Status			Type of family			Education								Occupation						
Family No.	Head of the family	Total family members	Family Member No.	Infant (1-12 months)	Under 5 (1-5 years)	School going (6-12 yr)	Adolescent (13-17 yr)	Early Adult (18-45 yrs)	Late Adults (46-59 yrs)	Geriatric (60 yr and above)	Male	Female	Transgender	Hindu	Muslim	Christian	Sikh	Others	General	OBC	SC	ST	Married	Unmarried/Single	Widow	Nuclear	Joint	Separated	Illiterate	Able to read and write	Primary	Secondary	Graduate	Postgraduate	Others	Unemployed	Housewife	Govt. job	Private job	Retired	Daily wage worker	Total family income (₹)

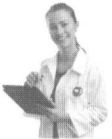

2.2 HOUSING STANDARDS

Family No.	Ownership of house		Type of house			No. of rooms in house	Bathroom					Latrine					Electricity		Water supply				Kitchen			Type of fuel used				
	Own	Rented	Pucca	Semi pucca	Kuccha		Not Available	Available Own	Available Public	Hygienic	Unhygienic	Not Available	Available Own	Available Public	Hygienic	Unhygienic	Available	Not available	Tap	Well	Lake/pond	Others	Separate	Corner of room	Others	LPG	Electricity	Kerosene	Wood	Others

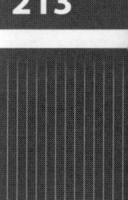

2.3 HOUSING ENVIRONMENT AND SANITATION

Family No.	Modern sanitation facility		Drainage system		Refuse disposal					Domestic animal (If present)						Cattle shed		Domestic birds/poultry (If present)			Poultry shed		Rodents (If present)		Insects (If present)				Street animals (If present)			
	Drainage system	Sewage system	Closed	Open	Open dumping	Composting	Burning	Community bins	Municipality collection	Dog	Cats	Buffalo	Cow	Goat	Others	Yes	No	Hen/cock	Parrot	Others	Yes	No	Rat	Others	Mosquitoes	Flies	Ticks	Others	Dogs	Cats	Cows	Others

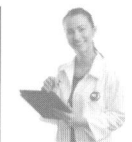

2.4 FAMILY PLANNING AND COMMON HEALTH PROBLEMS

Family No.	Total no. of eligible couple in the family	Total no. of women (15-49 years) in the family	Eligible Couple No./ Name	Method adopted for family planning								Family Member No.	Common health problems in last one year (Mention the number from the list given below)						Events within the last one year						
				Not using any method	Temporary methods					Permanent methods			Communicable disease *	Non-Communicable disease**	Nutritional problems***	Mental health problems#	Acute problems##	Chronic problems###	Any Birth	Any Death	Any neonatal death (infant less than 7 days)	Any neonate death (infant less than 28 days)	Any maternal death during antenatal, childbirth and postnatal period due to complications	Any Stillbirth	Any infant death
					Condom	Oral pill	Copper-T	Injectable	Sub-dermal implants	Tubectomy	Vasectomy														

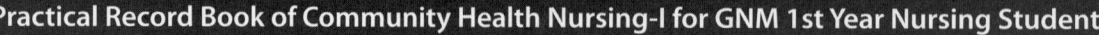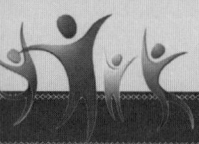

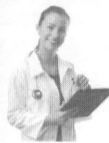

Common Health Problems

*Communicable disease –
1. Respiratory infection
2. Meningitis
3. Tuberculosis
4. Viral hepatitis
5. Diarrhea
6. Typhoid
7. Dengue
8. Malaria
9. Filaria
10. Viral infection
11. Others, specify _____

**Noncommunicable disease –
1. Stroke
2. Anaemia
3. Hypertension
4. Diabetes mellitus
5. Cardiovascular diseases
6. Cancer
7. Obesity
8. Others, specify _____

***Nutritional Problems-
1. Malnutrition
   (a) Over nutrition
   (b) Under nutrition
   (c) Other Nutritional deficiencies

#Mental Illness-
1. Depression
2. Mania
3. BPAD
4. Schizophrenia
5. OCD
6. Others, specify _____

##Acute Problems-
1. Cold
2. Cough
3. Pain
4. Inflammation/edema
5. Cut/bruises
6. Strain
7. Others, specify _____

###Chronic Problems-
1. COPD
2. Asthma
3. Rheumatic heart disease
4. Arthritis
5. Diabetes mellitus
6. Cancer
7. Hypertension
8. Others, specify _____

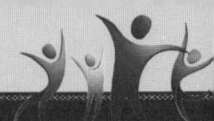

Family Folder (Sample Proforma)

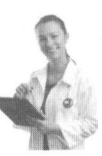

Name and Address of Institute: _____

DEMOGRAPHIC PROFILE

Village/Area: _____ Tehsil/Taluka: _____ Block: _____
District: _____ SC: _____ PHC: _____ CHC: _____

FAMILY PROFILE

Name of Head of the Family: _____
Address: _____
_____
Religion—Hindu/Muslims/Sikh/Christian/Others: _____
_____
Caste—GEN/SC/ST/OBC: _____
Language known: Hindi/English/Others: _____
_____

Family Type: Nuclear/Joint: _____
Family Size (Total Members): _____
Ownership of House: Own/Rented: _____
Occupation of the head of the family: Unemployed/ Government/Private Job/Self-Employed/daily wage worker/ homemaker/others: _____
Total Monthly Family Income ₹: _____
Per Capita Family Income ₹: _____

FAMILY COMPOSITION AND CHARACTERISTICS

S. No.	Name of the family members	Relationship with head of the family	Date of Birth/ Sex (Male-M/ Female-F/ Transgender-T)	Marital Status (Unmar-ried/Mar-ried)	Educa-tional status	Occu-pation	Monthly income (₹)	Dietary habits (Veg/ Non-veg)	Addiction (smoking alcohol/ drugs/ others)	Health status (Healthy/ un-healthy)
1.										
2.										
3.										
4.										
5.										
6.										
7.										
8.										
9.										
10.										

HOUSING STANDARDS AND ENVIRONMENTAL CONDITIONS

Characteristic	Parameters
Type of house	Pucca/Semi pucca/Katcha
Site	Elevated from surroundings/depressed from surroundings
Total number of living room	1/2/3/4/5/6/7/8/ _____
Space per person	Adequate (1 room -2 persons, 2 rooms -3 persons, 3 rooms – 5 persons, 4 rooms -7 persons, 5 or more rooms - 10 persons (additional 2 for each further room Inadequate (if above criteria is not fulfilled)

contd…

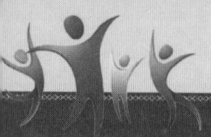
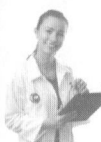

Characteristic	Parameters
Ventilation	Adequate (doors and windows facing each other in each room)
	Inadequate (doors and windows not facing each other in each room)
Bathroom	Not available/If available—Own/Public
Hygiene	Hygienic/Unhygienic
Wall	Plastered or Cemented/Tiled/Wooden/Unplastered/Mud//Others, specify _____
Roof	
Height	Less than 10 feet/More than 10 feet
Painting	Light colored/Dark colored
Day light	Adequate (Able to read the small fonts of newspaper inside the room during the day without any artificial lighting)
	Inadequate (Not able to read the small fonts of newspaper inside the room during the day without any artificial lighting)
Latrine	Not available/If available—Own/Public
Hygiene	Hygienic/Unhygienic
Electricity	Not available/Available
Drinking water supply	Tap/Well/Lake/Pond/Others, specify _____
Kitchen	Separate/Corner of the room/Others, specify _____
Type of fuel used	LPG/Electricity/Kerosene/Wood/Others, specify _____
Open space around the house	Absent/Present
Stagnant water around the house	Absent/Present
Street road	Tar/Cement/Mud/Others
Street light	Absent/Present
Modern sanitation facility	
Drainage system	Yes/No
Sewage system	Yes/No
Drainage System	Closed/Open
Refuse Disposal	Open dumping/Composting/Burning/Municipality collection/Community bins/Others, specify _____
Domestic animal	Absent/If present—Dog/Cow/Buffalo/Goat/Camel/Others, specify _____
Separate cattle shed (for the house with domestic animals)	Yes/No
Domestic birds/Poultry	Absent/If present—Hen/Cock/Parrot/Others, specify _____
Separate poultry shed/cage (for the house with domestic birds)	Yes/No
Rodents	Absent/If present—Rat/Others, specify _____
Street animals	Absent/If present—Dogs/Cats/Cows/Others, specify _____
Insect vectors	Absent/If present—Mosquitoes/Flies/Ticks/Others, specify _____

SOCIOECONOMIC STATUS

Social class/Socioeconomic status (according to rural/urban socioeconomic scale)
....

VULNERABLE/TARGET GROUPS IN THE FAMILY

Total eligible couples _____   Children (0–1 years) _____   Adolescent Girls _____

Total postnatal mothers _____   Children (1–3 years) _____   Elderly (above 60 years) _____

Total antenatal mothers _____   Children (3–5 years) _____   Other, specify _____

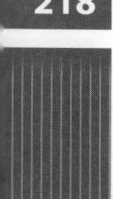

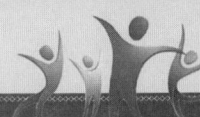
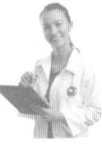

FAMILY DIETARY PATTERN

Food group	Food item	Food consumption (Yes/No)	Frequency of consumption (servings per day or per week)	Method/Form of food preparation (boiling/steaming/raw/ pressure cooking/ frying/germination etc.)	Method of food storage at home (Hygienic-H/ Unhygienic-U)
Energy giving foods	Rice				
	Wheat				
	Tubers				
	Edible oil				
	Ghee				
	Butter				
Body building foods	Meat				
	Fish				
	Poultry				
	Eggs				
	Pulses				
Protective foods	Vegetables				
	Fruits				
	Milk and milk products				
Beverages	Tea				
	Coffee				
	Water				
Others	Junk food				

FAMILY PLANNING STATUS (ELIGIBLE COUPLE)

S. No.	Name of the eligible couple (Mr. _____ Mrs_____)	Age (yrs.)/ Sex (Male-M Female-F)	Family planning practice Yes No	Temporary family planning method					Permanent family planning method		Month and year of adoption/ Duration of use
				Condom	Oral pills	Copper-T	Inject able	Implant	Tubectomy	Vasectomy	
1.											
2.											
3.											
4.											

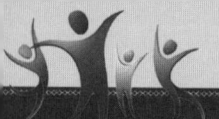 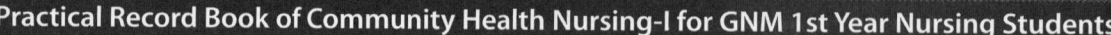

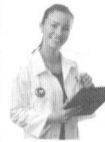

IMMUNIZATION STATUS

Age Group	Weeks/ Months/ Years	Current Vaccine Under UIP (2017)	Child Name/Vaccines/Date of administration (D.O.A.)					
			Child -1 _____		Child -2 _____		Child -3 _____	
			Vaccines	D.O.A.	Vaccines	D.O.A.	Vaccines	D.O.A.
Infant	At birth	BCG, OPV-0, Hep-B birth dose						
	6 weeks	OPV-1,Rota-1, Pentavalent-1, IPV-1, PCV-1						
	10 weeks	OPV-2,Rota-2, Pentavalent-2						
	14 weeks	OPV-3, Rota-3, Pentavalent-3, IPV-2, PCV-2						
	9 months	MR/Measles-1,Vit-A*, JE-1# PCV-Booster						
Under five Children	16–24 months	DPT-Booster-1, OPV-Booster, MR/Measles-2, JE-2#						
School Going	5–6 Years	DPT-Booster -2						
Adolescent	10 years	TT-1						
	16 years	TT-2						
Pregnancy		TT-1						
		TT-2						

*Vitamin A to be given every 6 months till five years of age and a separate chart is given below for documentation. #JE vaccine given in selected districts. **BCG:** Bacillus Calmette-Guerin; **Pentavalent [DPT:** diphtheria-pertussis-tetanus; **Hep B:** Hepatitis B; **Hib:**Haemophilus influenzae type b]; **JE:** Japanese Encephalitis; **MR/Measles/MMR:** Measles Mumps rubella; **OPV:** oral polio vaccine; **TT:** tetanus toxoid; **IPV:** inactivated poliovirus vaccine. **Rota-** Rotavirus vaccine, **PCV:** Pneumonia; Additional

Age (in months) →		9	18	24	30	36	42	48	54	60
	Dose →	1st	2nd	3rd	4th	5th	6th	7th	8th	9th
Vitamin-A Solution (D.O.A.)	Child-1 _____									
	Child-2 _____									
	Child-3 _____									

FAMILY HEALTH ASSESSMENT AND DOMICILIARY CARE

Date/Time	Assessment	Nursing Intervention	Evaluation	Signature	
				Student	Supervisor

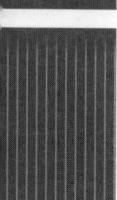

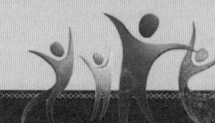
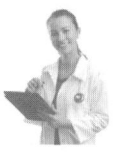

ANTHROPOMETRIC MEASUREMENTS

1. Weight

Average Birth-weight of Indian newborn is 2.7 to 2.9 kg .

Weight gain

In first 3 months = 25–30 gm/month

Then up to 1 year = 400 gms/month.

Note: In first 4–5 days after the birth, newborn babies loses their weight by 10%. From 10th day onwards, they regain their weight.

Usual weight gaining pattern

Age	Birth-weight
At birth	X
5 months	2X
1 year	3X
2 years	4X
3 years	5X
5 years	6X
7 years	7X
10 years	10X

Weight calculation

4-6 months = Birth-weight x 2

12 months = Birth-weight x 3

2 years = Birth-weight x 4

From 3–12 months = 1/2 (Age in months + 9) = Wt. in kg

1–6 years = Age in years x 2 + 8 = Wt. in kg

7–12 year = [Age in years x 7–5]/2 = Wt. in kg

For adult

According to Brocca Index

Expected weight = Height (in cm)-100 = Wt. in kg

2. Height

Usual height gaining pattern

Age	Length/height
At birth	50 cm
6 months	65 cm
1 year	75 cm
2 years	85 cm
3 years	95 cm
4 years	100 cm

Height calculation

From 2 to 12 years = Age (in years) x 6 + 77

After 4 years a child gains approximately 6 cm height every year until 12 years of age

3. Mid Arm Circumference (MAC)

Usual pattern of increase in mid arm circumference

Age	Mid arm circumference
At birth	11–12 cm
1 year	12–16 cm
1–5 years	16–17 cm
12 years	17–18 cm
15 years	20–21 cm

Classification of malnutrition (according to WHO)

Mid arm circumference	Grade
Above 13.5 cm	Normal
13.5–12.5 cm	Mild to Moderate(Grade- IandII)
Below 12.5 cm	Severe (Grade-III)

4. Head Circumference (HC)

It increases approximately 2 cm/month for first 3 months, 1 cm/month for next 3 months and 0.5 cm/month for rest of first year of life.

Usual pattern of increase in head circumference

Age	Head circumference
At birth	33–35 cm
3 months	40 cm
6 months	43 cm
2 years	48 cm
7 years	50 cm
12 years	52 cm
18 years	55 cm

Note: If there is 1 cm increase in head circumference in 2 weeks during first 3 months – Hydrocephalus is suspected.

5. Chest Circumference (CC)

Age	Chest circumference
At birth	2–3 cm less than Head Circumference (31–33 cm)
6–12 months	Both Chest Circumference and Head Circumference are equal
1 year	Chest Circumference >Head Circumference by 2.5 cm
5 years	Chest circumference is 5 cm>Head Circumference

6. Abdominal Circumference (AC)

Age	Abdominal circumference
At birth	32 cm

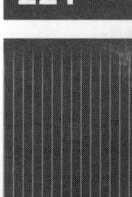

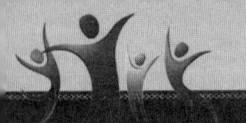
COMMUNITY PROFILE EVALUATION CRITERIA

Name of the Area _____ Date: _____

Maximum Marks 30

S. No.	Particulars	Marks Allotted	Obtained Marks
1.	Introduction	2	
2.	Health Care/NGO/Social/Religious facilities	2	
3.	Educational/Recreation/Communication/Transport facilities	2	
4.	Sociodemographic Data	2	
5.	Physical Characteristics of Area (Map)	2	
6.	Housing Standards	2	
7.	Housing Environment and Sanitation	2	
8.	Family Planning Status	2	
9.	Common Health Problems	2	
10.	Vital Statistics	2	
11.	Ongoing Community Health Programmes	2	
12.	Ongoing Social Welfare/Health Schemes	2	
13.	List of Community Leaders	2	
14.	Identified Community Health Needs	2	
15.	Community Health Action Plan	2	
	Total	**30**	

Remarks

_____

_____

_____

_____

_____

_____

Signature of Supervisor

Date

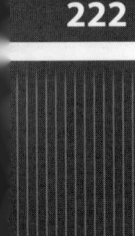

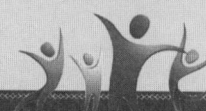

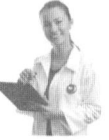

FAMILY NURSING CARE PLAN EVALUATION CRITERIA

Family Nursing Care Plan On _____ Date: _____

Maximum Marks 50

S. No.	Particulars	Marks Allotted	Obtained Marks
1.	Introduction	2	
2.	Family Composition and Family Characteristics	2	
3.	Family tree/Family Genogramme	2	
4.	Health Care/Social/Educational Facilities	2	
5.	Recreation/Communication/Transport/Religious facilities	2	
6.	Sketch of House	1	
7.	Housing Standard and Environmental Conditions	1	
8.	SOCIOECONOMIC STATUS	1	
9.	Vulnerable/Target Groups	1	
10.	Family Budget	1	
11.	Family Dietary Pattern	1	
12.	SOCIOCULTURAL ASPECTS	1	
13.	Family Planning Status	1	
14.	Immunization Status	1	
15.	Vital Events (Birth, Death, Marriage)	1	
16.	Family Health Profile	10	
17.	Health Need Identification/Prioritization/Nursing Diagnosis	4	
18.	Family Nursing Care Plan	12	
19.	Health Education	2	
20	References	2	
	Total	50	

Remarks

_____

_____

_____

_____

_____

Signature of Supervisor

Date

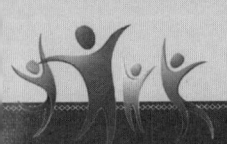
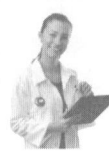

HEALTH ASSESSMENT EVALUATION CRITERIA

Health Assessment On: _____

Name of the Family Member: _____

Age/Sex: _____

Date: _____ Time: _____

Maximum Marks 40

S. No.	Particulars	Marks Allotted	Obtained Marks
1.	Identification data	1	
2.	History Collection	2	
3.	Family Composition and Characteristics	2	
4.	Family tree/Genogramme	1	
5.	Housing Standard and Environmental Conditions	2	
6.	Physical Examination/Assessment Skill	8	
7.	Lab Investigations	2	
8.	Medications	2	
9.	Dietary Pattern (24 Hours Recall)	2	
10.	Modified Diet Plan	2	
11.	Health Need-Identification/Prioritization/Nursing Diagnosis	3	
12.	Family Nursing Care Plan	8	
13.	Health Education	3	
14.	References	2	
	Total	**40**	

Remarks

_____

_____

_____

_____

_____

Signature of Supervisor

Date

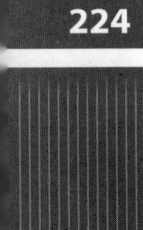

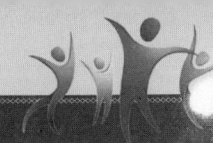

HEALTH EDUCATION EVALUATION CRITERIA

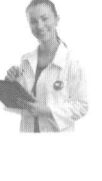

Health Education On: _____

Group: _____

Date: _____ Time: _____

Maximum Marks 30

S. No.	Particulars	Marks Allotted	Marks Obtained
1.	Selection of the Topic According to the Health/Group Need	2	
2.	Lesson Plan—Introduction	2	
3.	General and Specific Objectives	2	
4.	Content relevant to the topic	2	
5.	Content adequacy and sequence of organization	2	
6.	Incorporation of Research Input/Current trends/Issues	2	
7.	Summary and Conclusion	2	
8.	References	2	
9.	Classroom/sitting arrangement	2	
10.	Posture and Grooming (neat and tidy)	2	
11.	Communication Skills-language, voice audibility, clarity	2	
12.	Group Participation	2	
13.	Evaluation/feedback	2	
14.	Appropriate selection, preparation and use of A-V aid	2	
15.	Time coverage	2	
	Total	**30**	

Remarks

_____

_____

_____

_____

_____

Signature of Supervisor

Date

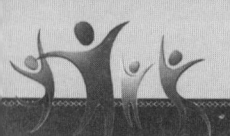

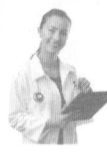

NUTRITIONAL ASSESSMENT (UNDER FIVE/ADULT) EVALUATION CRITERIA

Name of the Family Member: _____

Age/Sex: _____

Date: _____ Time: _____

Maximum Marks 30

S. No.	Particulars	Marks Allotted	Obtained Marks
1.	Identification data ,Family composition and characteristics	2	
2.	Anthropometric Measurements (including Growth chart plotting in Children)	4	
3.	Family Dietary Pattern	2	
4.	Assessment Skill for common nutritional deficiencies	4	
5.	Lab Investigations	2	
6.	Individual Dietary Pattern (24 Hours Recall)	3	
7.	Modified Diet Plan	3	
8.	Health Need-Identification/Prioritization/Nursing Diagnosis	3	
9.	Family Nursing Care Plan	5	
10.	Health Education and References	2	
	Total	**30**	

Remarks

_____

_____

_____

_____

_____

_____

_____

_____

_____

Signature of Supervisor

Date

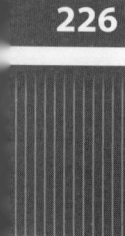

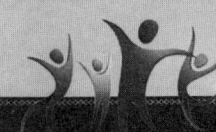

NUTRITIOUS FOOD PREPARATION/COOKING DEMONSTRATION EVALUATION CRITERIA

Cooking Demonstration On: _____

Name of the Family Member: _____

Age/Sex: _____

Date: _____ Time: _____

Maximum Marks 30

S. No.	Particulars	Good (3)	Average (2)	Poor (1)
1.	Develop the rapport with the family			
2.	Selection of demonstration according to nutritional need of the family member			
3.	Appropriate selection of ingredients and articles			
4.	Maintain hygiene (e.g. hand washing, cooking utensils)			
5.	Follow all the steps of preparation correctly			
6.	After care of the articles			
7.	Calculation of Nutritive value			
8.	Calculation of Price			
9.	Health education			
10.	Feed back from the family member			
	Total	30		

Remarks

_____

_____

_____

_____

_____

_____

_____

_____

Signature of Supervisor

Date

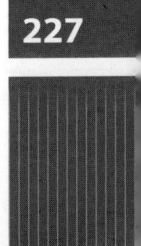

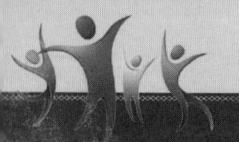

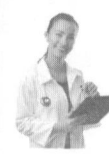

PROCEDURE EVALUATION CRITERIA

Bag Technique Procedure On _____ Date: _____

Maximum Marks 45

S. No.	Particulars	Good (3)	Average (2)	Poor (1)
1.	Develop the rapport with the family			
2.	Selection of procedure according to priority health need of the family			
3.	Preparation of community health bag according to the procedure			
4.	Follow bag technique correctly			
5.	Follow hand washing technique correctly			
6.	Preparation of the patient			
7.	Perform all the steps of procedure correctly			
8.	Carry out all the steps of procedure with scientific principles			
9.	Involvement of other family members in procedure			
10.	Communicate with patient and other family members while doing procedure			
11.	After care of the patient			
12.	After care of the articles and the community health bag			
13.	Dispose the waste correctly			
14.	Health education after the procedure			
15	Documentation of the procedure			
	Total	45		

Remarks

_____
_____
_____
_____
_____
_____
_____
_____
_____

Signature of Supervisor

Date

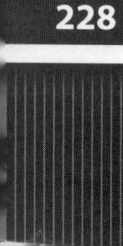

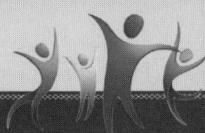

PREPARATION OF AUDIO-VISUAL AIDS EVALUATION CRITERIA

Topic: _____

Maximum Marks 20

S. No.	Particulars	Marks Allotted	Marks Obtained
1.	Plan for A-V aid Preparation- Introduction, definition, objectives, principles, steps, layout, references	5	
2.	Principles followed	2	
3.	Budget calculation/Economical	2	
4.	Appropriate use of material and articles for model preparation	2	
5.	Accuracy/Size according to given dimensions	2	
6.	Utility	2	
7.	Simplicity	1	
8.	Solidity	1	
9.	Creativity	1	
10.	Submission on time	2	
	Total	**20**	

Remarks

_____
_____
_____
_____
_____
_____
_____
_____

Signature of Supervisor

Date

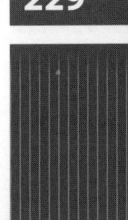

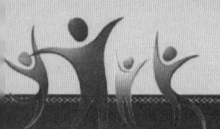

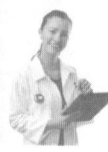

HEALTH ACTIVITY/CLINIC/CAMP EVALUATION CRITERIA

Health Activity/Clinic/Camp On _____

Date: _____   Time: _____

Place: _____

Maximum Marks 20

S. No.	Particulars	Marks Allotted	Obtained Marks
1.	Introduction/Objectives/Purpose	2	
2.	Arrangement of equipment and resources and their source	2	
3.	Health personnel involvement/their function	2	
4.	Map/floor plan showing arrangement of stations/equipment/resources	2	
5.	Organization of activities at different stations as per participant's need	2	
6.	Active participation in different activities of clinic/camp	2	
7.	Maintenance of record and report	2	
8.	Discipline/Time management	2	
9.	Evaluation and feedback from the participant	2	
10.	Student Learning	2	
	Total	**20**	

Remarks

_____

_____

_____

_____

_____

_____

_____

_____

_____

Signature of Supervisor

Date

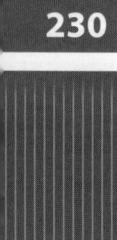

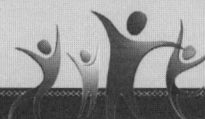

OBSERVATION VISIT EVALUATION CRITERIA

Place of Visit: _____ Date: _____

Address: _____

Maximum Marks 20

S. No.	Particulars	Marks Allotted	Obtained Marks
1.	Introduction	2	
2.	Visit Objectives/Purpose	2	
3.	Organization Structure/Staffing Pattern	2	
4.	Lay out of Physical Set-up	2	
5.	Welfare Activities/functions of Organization	2	
6.	Source of Funding/Budgeting	2	
7.	Record and report maintained	2	
8.	Student participation in the visit	2	
9.	Discipline/Time management	2	
10.	Student's learning from the visit	2	
	Total	20	

Remarks

_____

_____

_____

_____

_____

_____

_____

_____

_____

Signature of Supervisor

Date

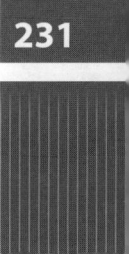

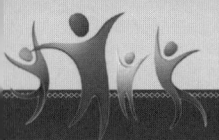

FAMILY FOLDER/HEALTH RECORD EVALUATION CRITERIA

Family Folder No: _____

Name of the Head of the Family: _____

Address: _____

Maximum Marks 10

S. No.	Particulars	Marks Allotted	Marks Obtained
1.	Clear	1	
2.	Accurate	1	
3.	Relevant	1	
4.	Completeness	1	
5.	Uniform writing style	1	
6.	Grammar/sentence formation	1	
7.	Up-to-date	1	
8.	Signed with date and time	1	
9.	Neat	1	
10.	Properly kept in folder cover or file	1	
	Total	**10**	

Remarks

_____

_____

_____

_____

_____

_____

_____

_____

Signature of Supervisor

Date

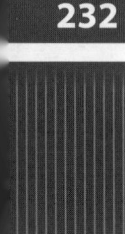

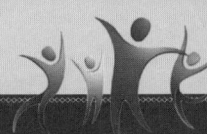

Bibliography

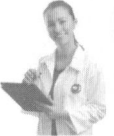

1. Santhi MV. Practical Record Book of Community Health Nursing –I. 1st edition. New Delhi:CBS Publisher and Distributors Pvt. Ltd; 2016.

2. Gulani KK. Community Health Nursing (Principles & Practices) 2nd edition. Delhi. Kumar Publishing House, 2005.

3. Singh MK. Complete Review of Preventive and Social Medicine. 2nd edition. New Delhi: CBS Publisher and Distributors Pvt. Ltd; 2016.

4. Park. K. Parks Text Book of Preventive and Social Medicine. 23rd edition: Jabalpur (MP). M/s Banarsidas Bhanot; 2015.

5. Taylor CR, Lillis C, LeMone P, Lynn P. Fundamentals of Nursing. The Art and Science of Nursing Care. 7th edition. New Delhi: Wolters Kluwer (India) Pvt. Ltd; 2012.

6. Sr. Nancy. Stephanie's Principles and Practice of Nursing. 6th edition. Indore (MP). NR Publishing House; 2016.

7. Rana AK, Saini SK. Practical Record Book of Midwifery. 1st edition. New Delhi: CBS Publisher and Distributors Pvt. Ltd; 2016.

8. Babu M, Gusain S. Clinical Case Record for Midwives. 4th edition. Delhi. Kumar Publishing House; 2009.

9. Government of India. Ministry of Health & Family Welfare. Guidelines for antenatal care and skilled attendance at birth by ANMs and LHVs-2010. [online] Available from: www.nhp.gov.in/sites/default/files/anm_guidelines. pdf [Assessed Sep 15, 2016]

10. Singh T et al. Socioeconomic status scales updated for 2017. Int J Res Med Sci. 2017;5(7):3264-3267 [online] Available from: www.msjonline.org [Assessed July 29, 2017]

11. Dutta P. Pediatric Nursing. 2nd edition. New Delhi: Jaypee Brothers Medical Publishers; 2009.

12. Sudhakar A. Practical Record Book of Child Health Nursing. 1st edition. New Delhi: CBS Publisher and Distributors Pvt. Ltd; 2016.

13. Gupta P. Clinical Methods in Pediatrics. 2nd edition. New Delhi: CBS Publisher and Distributors Pvt. Ltd; 2011.

14. Marlow DR, Redding BA. Textbook of Pediatric Nursing. South Asian edition. New Delhi. Elsevier India Private Limited; 2013.

15. World Health Organization. Guidelines for the implementation of the health promoting schools initiative (HPSI).Brazzaville-Congo: [online] Available from: URL: www.afro.who.int/[Assessed on 2012 Dec 12]

16. Nettina SM. Lippincott Manual of Medical and Surgical Nursing. 8th edition. New Delhi: Wolters Kluwer (India) Pvt Ltd; 2006.

17. Sharma R. Practical Record Book of Medical Surgical Nursing-II. 1st edition. New Delhi: CBS Publisher and Distributors Pvt. Ltd; 2016.

18. Singh R. Food and Nutrition for Nurses (B.Sc. Nursing). 1st edition. New Delhi: Jaypee Brothers Medical Publishers; 2012.

19. Budhwar S. A Textbook of Food and Nutrition for Nurses. 1st edition. Delhi. Kumar Publishing House, 2015.

Notes

Notes

Notes